Just Call Me Dean

And Don't Rain on My Parade

Florene Stewart Poyadue
(Via Dean A. A. Poyadue)

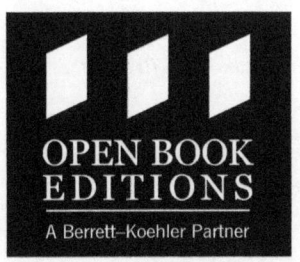

OPEN BOOK
EDITIONS
A Berrett–Koehler Partner

Just Call Me Dean
And Don't Rain on my Parade

iUniverse books may be ordered through booksellers or by contacting:

iUniverse
1663 Liberty Drive
Bloomington, IN 47403
www.iuniverse.com
1-800-Authors (1-800-288-4677)

ISBN: 978-1-4620-3431-4 (sc)
ISBN: 978-1-4620-3432-1 (e)
ISBN: 978-1-4620-3430-7 (dj)

Library of Congress Control Number: 2011916252

Printed in the United States of America

iUniverse rev. date: 10/25/2011

Dedicated to:

Dean and Kim

All who seek a full, happy, interdependent way of life

CONTENTS

Acknowledgments

Of course, without Dean A. A. Poyadue, this book would not exist. He has hounded me to write it since he was about twenty years old; he is now thirty-five. And if he did not have the strength, wisdom, fortitude, and courage to face life and take on its challenges, there would be no words to print—no uplifting story to tell, no very "special" everyday hero to capture our imagination and our hearts.

Dean wanted me to put his story onto paper, from his unique, understated, and sometimes somewhat-lopsided point of view. By forcing myself to commit to time at my computer, by calling on him for clarifications where my memory failed, and by reviewing drafts with him, I believe we have pulled it off.

I always have to acknowledge the huge contribution to any of my endeavors that is made by my soul mate, my spouse for over fifty years, Octave A. Poyadue (better known as Sweetie). And I extend this gratitude also to our other three children, Turhan Michael, Keith Matthew, and Jill Alexandria; as well as to our seven grandchildren, Jay Quinn, Antonia Symone, Aidan Gabriel, Tayelor Marie, Griffin Matthew, Mira Alexandria, and Asher Gabriel. They all make my life one that is not only fulfilled, but also filled full of priceless moments. Because of their precious time and attention to my endeavors, I am able to write, to work, and to perform acts of kindness in the community. They listen to and provide ideas, read drafts, remind me of our wonderful and complicated family history, provide the love and hugs that make life meaningful, and inspire me to get on with the work of writing, and much more.

I thank the many friends and families of children with special needs who read and added thoughts along the way. I will not start to name them individually, as I will surely forget someone and then get myself into a lot of trouble. You guys all know who you are and how much I love you and appreciate what you have done.

A very special thank you goes to Dean's wife, Kim, who prodded me to "Get on with it!" And when Kim gives an order, people usually listen; I know I do. Thanks Kim, for the gentle word shove.

Dean would not have been able to have the life experience that he has had without a nonprofit organization called Parents Helping Parents (PHP). Its mission is to ensure that children with special needs reach their full potential and receive appropriate health care, education, and services by providing them: well-informed families, dedicated professionals, and responsive service systems. While I founded PHP, I also fully and often used PHP to acquire services and enhance Dean's life. *PHP is all about building bright futures for children with special needs.* If you have a child with special needs, I hope there is a parent-directed family resource center in your community. If there is not a center in your area, why not start one? Hint – Just Google Parents Helping Parents – San Jose, CA.; and also get a copy of The Parent to Parent Handbook by Santelli, Poyadue, and Young (2001) Baltimore: Paul H. Brookes Publishing.

Without Dean's rich life experiences, this book could not have been written. Thanks, Dean, for being a "can do" (or an "at least, will try") kind of guy. You are a guy willing to take on the challenges of the world—with a smile.

To my iUniverse editors, coordinators, consultants, and other literary guides, I offer my sincere thanks for your support and forward movement of this very personal project. Your assistance, time, and expertise allowed me to fulfill a fervent commitment to someone very special in my life. You also allowed me to give a mighty shout out to a whole community of warm, wonderful, contributing young adults with special needs whom I admire and wish a lifetime of opportunities, love, and possibilities. As this book works its way across the nation, and into the hearts of America, those with any kind of difference will forever be singing your praise for bringing this quality product forth.

I must give a big shout out of thanks to my three computer assistance gurus—husband Octave, son Keith for being my performance coach, and especially grandson Jay Quinn for truly being my computer 'guide at the side'.

A very big final thank you is sent out to all my extended family members (Dean's aunts, uncles, cousins, in-laws, godparents) and the many friends and professionals throughout California and the nation who have positively contributed so much to Dean's successful life. You will read about some of them in this book, but due to time and space limits, many are not mentioned in the book; their contributions are no less important to Dean and me. We both send a heartfelt thank you, thank you, many thanks to you all!

Yes, it does "take a village." But then again, the village has gained as well.

PREFACE

One day when Dean and his dad were 'reviewing his past,' as they so often did; they had the following, very poignant conversation:

"Dad, did you take me to Disneyland?"
"Yes, I did. Do you remember it, Dean?"
"No, Dad. Dad, did you take me to Yosemite?"
"Yes, Dean, I did. Do you remember that?"
"No, Dad. Dad, did you take me to NASA?"
"Oh, yes, Dean. Do you remember that?"
"No, Dad."
"My gosh, Dean, I wasted my money."
"Oh, no, Dad, *it's all a part of me!*"

So much of what happens to us, whether we remember it very well or not at all, makes its mark on us. Dean has so wisely figured out that it becomes a part of who we are and how we function in life—for better or for worse. That is a great "truth" to know. Dean knows that truth, thanks to his dad and the adventures he provided. Dean also knows that he is a more grateful person, a more self-assured guy, and a more courageous man because of those wonderful, positive life experiences his wonderful father provided.

Won't you come along on the uplifting voyage of his life? You will travel a bit back in time and then move rapidly forward through the unique experiences of a successful young man, a young man whose journey through life allows us to appreciate the wonders of accomplishing simple, everyday tasks, as he takes on and meets the challenges that assail and the opportunities that beckon him. His name is Dean Archibald Anthony Poyadue, and he was born with Down syndrome*.

Dean's story will introduce you to the "up" side of Down. Yes, there can be another side, but you will have to read his mom's story or other books written on the subject to experience that down side. You are encouraged not to rain on Dean's parade, but instead, join him in his positive approach to moving forward in life. Try it; you might like to use it for your own life as well and find it beneficial for your growth, health, and happiness. It won't cost you much more than a positive attitude and a smile.

Dean is not alone in his success. Many others with a variety of special needs or disabilities have traveled successful roads of life. We salute them all. We applaud their contributions to the success and pleasantness of our planet. Like the young man who lost his eyesight but became a great sculptor; he said that he would not have his vision back, if he had to give up all he had gained since he lost it.

Most parents of children with special needs will tell you that they spend an awesome amount of time with their children, getting to know and understand their needs, their desires, their disability, and *especially* their abilities. Sometimes, they feel as though they are joined to their child at the head or heart, if not the hip. In that context, this book is written by Dean's mom but from the perspective of his thoughts, actions, words, and reactions (behavioral and emotional) to events in his life. Any liberties that are taken with words or expressions is done to simply get his side of the story out and to enhance the reader's comprehension.

This book will cover the major aspects of Dean's life: his birth, his family, neighborhood integration; a very special lifelong friendship with a 'regular' kid, and his education, which consisted of early infant stimulation, preschool, Head Start, elementary school, junior high, high school, and college. It also contains information about his health, friends, awards, sports, siblings, and fun activities like dating, dancing, bowling, and the excitement of being behind the wheel of a moving car. Of course, his life's history would not be complete without a look at his transition to independent living, his bachelor days, religious activities, service agencies that support the many aspects of his life, his gainful employment, and of course his marriage to the beautiful Kimberly.

If you have someone in your family who has special needs, you will find this book uplifting. It may provide information or resources perhaps previously unknown or unfamiliar to you. If you do not have a person with special needs in your life, here is a significant opportunity to broaden your knowledge of the world you live in, to take a peek into the world of disability or special needs, and to grow as a caring and interested, as well as interesting, human being. This book has been written especially for you, to increase your comfort with millions of your fellow Americans who have a special need or disability.

If you are a professional who works with individuals with special needs, this short story can show you the other side of the coin. A professional who may have worked many years in the field, and suddenly finds him or herself the parent of a child with special needs, often gets a rather rude awakening to what the world of disability is all about. Their eyes are suddenly opened to what families are experiencing on the other side of the school table or hospital bed. This little book can help provide that awakening without your having to give birth to a child with special needs.

Dean has told his mom more than once, "It's my life," so let us get started on the life, times, and philosophies of Dean A. A. Poyadue.

*Down syndrome is a chromosome abnormality wherein the person so affected is born with three chromosomes on the twenty-first pair of chromosomes instead of the usual two. This extra chromosome can cause a number of physical and intellectual changes.

FLEETING MOMENT

Sometimes when I just glimpse my son,
I see,
The little ole boy
That was to be.
DAMN CHROMOSOME!

Three years have flown,
For you and me.
And now, with wiser eyes
I see.
You are the boy that was to be.
WELCOME HOME!!!!!

—Florene Stewart Poyadue

This poem is dedicated to all parents, especially those who just happen to have a child with special needs.

All children will benefit, and all children are valuable.

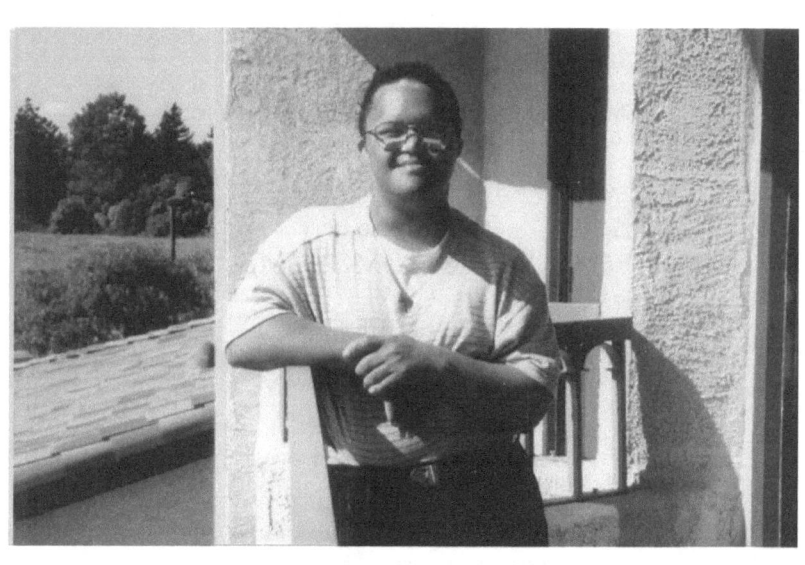

An Introduction

A Reason For Call Me Dean...

Beyond hoping to make a living, or at least add to their income, most writers no doubt have at least two or three major reasons for spending numerous hours of valuable time creating that all important, unique item we call a book. Sometimes, as with a Huckelberry Finn or To Kill a Mocking Bird, the book takes on a significance and purpose far beyond the author's original intensive purposes.

Both of the aforementioned books either surreptitiously, in spite of, or because of their simplicity of story and approach, helped define eras in a great country's history. They heightened awareness of racial issues, and continue to be used as tools for teaching the power of truth, tolerance, love, friendship and commitment to right over might, wrong thinking, and/or injustice.

My dream is that this memoir Just Call Me Dean... an unassuming and overwhelmingly positive story of a child overcoming intellectual and speech deficits, while lacking-in-dialogue presentation, will effect in a positive way our thinking and behavior towards individuals with 'a difference.' That difference may be disability, race, gender, sexual orientation, skin color, land of origin, religion or any other attribute. "Dean" expects to cast a broad outreach net.

Who is included in this outreach? I'm glad that you asked the question. It includes:

- The general population of our country which is probably not aware that a recent Gallup survey finds that this country is not as accepting of people with intellectual disabilities as many European nations
- Parents of all children (particularly those who have children with special needs) who want the best possible outcomes for their offspring,
- And helping professionals (teachers, nurses, physicians, numerous therapists), and paraprofessionals, including those learning their chosen fields, who are involved in the lives of individuals who may need assistance

How many of us realize that there are millions of Americans with disabilities? Not just children born with birth defects but also those injured on sports fields, in accidents on our highways, our military heroes on battle fields of war, and those affected by numerous diagnoses such as multiple sclerosis, muscular dystrophy, Lou Gherigs disease, and arthritis that can strike the very young as well as the old, just to name a few. The rise in autism is often called 'epidemic'; and schools have numerous students who have some type of learning disability (dyslexia, dysgraphia, ADD ADHD.) This is just a part of the list.

Positive changes expected from reading Dean... include: broadening our expectations of ourselves first, other adults and children, especially those who have a special need, and giving challenged children a chance to try, and to show what they can or can not do. If Dean causes even one family just leaving the hospital with a newborn with special needs, to bond and fall in love with their child, and to go beyond just accepting, but appreciating the unique individual they have, and the gifts they can bring; or if one professional broadens his or her approach as they interact with such families, thus becoming a good role model for others— writing Dean will have been well worth every hour given it.

When the world thought that you would never even learn to tie your shoes, and you grow up and tie the knot, go to college, hold a meaningful job, write your own checks to pay your rent—that is a big deal. Ordinary accomplishments become major reasons for excitement. It is important for the world to know it, and it is exceedingly important for the next 'guy with a difference' that the world encounters to know it, if he or she is to be given a fair chance at a full and inclusive life.

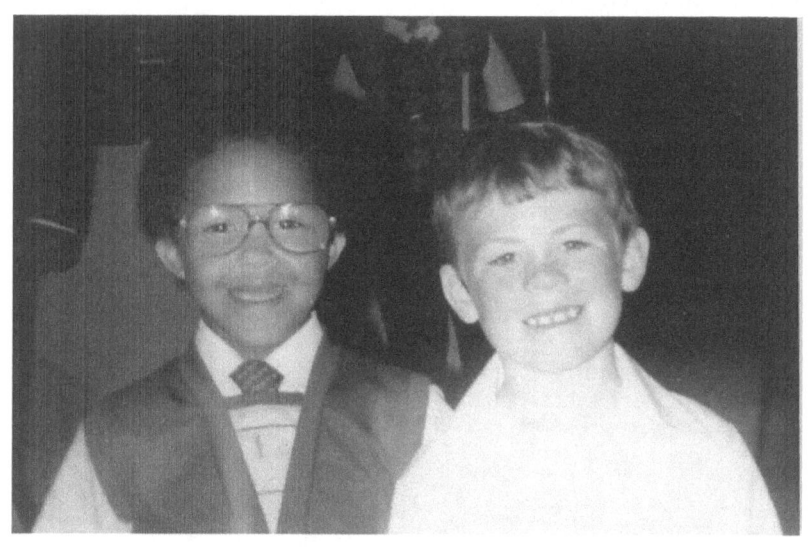

Chapter 1
0–6 Years of Age

In the Beginning ...

I know that ladies do not like to talk about their birthdays, but my mom was forty-one years old when I was born. And if I had just waited seven more days inside of her, my birth date would have been the same as Mom and Dad's wedding anniversary. I think that would have been cool. But instead of crashing in on September 30, their very special day, I was born on September 23, 1975.

My dad named me Dean. I later learned that he had a lot of respect for two guys who were named Dean: Dean Rusk, who was secretary of state under President John F. Kennedy and President Lyndon B. Johnson, and Dean Atcheson, secretary of state under President Harry S. Truman. You can tell my dad knew from the beginning that I was going to be an important guy. My mom insisted on adding her father's name, Archibald, as my middle name because she said that he was a "can do" type of guy. The Catholic priest who christened me added the name Anthony, for that saint who is well known in the church. Not that I am a saint, mind you, but I had to have a saint's name attached to me according to Catholic traditions. Why didn't the priest just use Archibald?

During my christening ceremony, the priest said, "I am not sure that there is a Saint Archibald."

My mom feigned disappointment at the news, as she said, "Do you imply my dear departed father is not a saint?"

The priest made no reply; he just gave a weak smile and continued, "What other saint's name would you like?"

My dad stated proudly but matter-of-factly, "My middle name is Anthony." So, I am called Dean Archibald Anthony Poyadue, a name that I really like. I always try to remember to put my double A's in the middle whenever I am signing anything ... Dean A. A. Poyadue.

And yet, I do have one little regret: I wish they could have found it in their naming ritual to include "Salvadore." Now that is another great sounding name. I like it a lot, and it belonged to my other grandfather. I am very much into "family and traditions," so this will not be the last time Mom and Dad will hear, "Why don't I have Salvadore in my name?" Oh well, I had learned a good lesson early in life: you can't always "have it your way," as is promised at some fast food restaurants.

Now that I was older and had an official name like my sister and brothers before me, Mom took me to the neighbors' homes to introduce me as her "new bundle of joy." She told me that she spent some time on how that introduction would be played out. She settled on just saying, "This is my new son, Dean." She thought that since she did not use an adjective when introducing her last baby ("This is Jill, my genius"), she would not do so when introducing me (such as, "This is Dean, my Downs").

So I was introduced as simply Dean. Mom was determined that I was to be a part of the neighborhood and an integral part of, but not the whole heart of, the family. And if the neighbors or friends had any questions, my mom was eager to educate them all about Down syndrome, starting with the fact that there is no *s* on the word *Down*. The physician who identified this syndrome was Dr. Charles Langdon Down, and it is named after him.

About two or three months after my birth, Mom bumped into

my pediatrician at the grocery store one day, and he gave her some "exciting" news as we were leaving. He said something like, "Blah, blah, blah … the test was positive, he does have Down syndrome/Trisomy 21. It is just plain Trisomy 21, not Mosaic Downs, or any abnormality of the parents' chromosomes. It just happens."

Mom quietly said, "Thanks," and we quickly headed for our car in the parking lot.

My mom is smart, and she's a nurse; so I think she already knew that "exciting" news report before the doctor told her. She seemed to take that "positive" test result as a sign to positively get started to work on my education. While my brothers and sister started school at about three years of age, I was enrolled in an Early Infant Stimulation class before I was three months old. I was so young that, of course I needed a parent right there in class with me. It seems that mom *wanted* to learn, as much as I *needed* to learn.

Did the doctors, nurses, and social workers tell my family about that early intervention program? Not really. My parents learned about it from other parents who had children with special needs. Alex's mom and John's mom told my mom about the class when they were at a parent support group meeting.

Alex's mom and John's mom seemed to know a lot about what was available to help me learn and grow. They seemed happy and eager to tell my mom all they knew. They explained that the Infant Stimulation class consisted of six to ten parents. The parents were almost always moms—not that dads could not come if they wanted. The class meetings were held at the home of one of the participating parents of a child with special needs.

The children had all kinds of special needs such as spina bifida, cerebral palsy, hydrocephalous, and other developmental disabilities. Some of them had become disabled through injury. And some of them were having problems, but they had no specific diagnosis. Parents of children in this last group seemed to have more concerns, confusion, and anger than many of the other parents. Many parents in this last group said that it was worse for them not having a specific diagnosis from which to plan for the future, or proceed with care and interventions for their children. Some said that there was just something very frustrating about "not knowing." For them, not having a name to attach to their child's problem had become a major problem itself.

Like the other kids (actually babies), I sat on Mom's lap, as she sat in a circle on the floor with the other parents and professional helpers at our Infant Stimulation class (it was also called "Atypical Infant Motivation"). They sang songs to us, exercised and massaged our arms and legs, or performed whatever activity was appropriate for helping the individual child progress or improve. They discussed all kinds of issues: health care, education, their feelings, concerns for spouses, our brothers and sisters and the rest of the family, our progress (or lack thereof), and services available. They were especially interested in discussing those services and cures that were *not* available that they so strongly wished for. They learned how to strengthen our bodies and minds, and perhaps to strengthen their own. These were parents helping each other, while helping us kids as well.

I have often heard Mom say that parents need to take care of themselves and their relationship with each other as one of the first steps to taking good care of their children. She would say that the mom and dad are like the trunk of a tree, which must be strong if it is to support the branches, which are the children, and different problems the family might face.

One of the hardest things these parents had to get comfortable with was the idea that their child's condition was something that was not going to get all better and go away. Many professionals also have trouble coping with the fact that while they may have a diagnosis for their patient or client, there is no prescription they can provide that will cure it. This is going to be lifelong—ongoing—forever. Even *I* had to learn this. You will see me confront this issue a bit later. Just keep reading.

A social worker with a master's degree (MSW) and an occupational therapist (OT) conducted the Infant Stimulation program for an agency called Hope. Isn't that a neat name for the agency helping us? The OT concentrated on the kids' needs. Meanwhile, the MSW concentrated on the parents' needs. The morning hours went by quickly. We attended this training and therapy class once or twice a week.

Before we knew it, I was off of Mom's lap and walking by twelve months of age. Wow! My first big accomplishment; medical books say it takes some of us kids two or three years to learn to walk. By fourteen months of age, they kicked me out of Early Infant Stimulation and moved me up to the special school for eighteen-month-old kids. I was on a roll, four whole months ahead of my time schedule.

There were only six kids in this new class. What a lucky day for me! We had a teacher, two teacher's aides, as well as a speech therapist and a psychologist on special days. This was really good—it was one-on-one care and training most of the time. The staff's philosophy was to expect that we could master some, if not all, normal behavior if they presented information in the right way, presented it often enough, and presented it with added rewards. The goal for us kids was to reach for the norm, and the staff's goal was to maintain their high expectation that we could learn. It was amazing how well it worked.

Thank goodness they did not accept or teach to abnormal behavior. I think they realized that if they did not offer age appropriate goals, we could not even venture into that more "normal" realm of behavior. Our teachers needed to expect us to learn, in order for us to have a good chance at learning.

Probably, all teachers need to believe in their students' ability to learn, if the students are to do their best and reach their full potential.

In this class, I had my first real teacher. Teacher Pat was great! She became a true friend of the family—attending my birthday parties, helping my mom create a parent-to-parent organization called Parents Helping Parents, as well as writing notes back and forth to my family about what I was doing in class. These notes also explained what my family should work on in order to help me reach my next milestone or developmental goals (physical development, speech, toilet training, and everything else).

You will hear more about Teacher Pat as you read on. For example, much later, when I graduated from high school, she was right there to celebrate with us. Can you believe it? It has been over thirty years, and she is still in my life, cheering me on!

I learned so much from Teacher Pat about making sounds, saying words, raising my hand to take turns, working with special toys, potty training, learning sign language, feeding myself, and a lot of other things. Actually, I learned so much that by three years of age, I was moved up to a Head Start class. My family was so proud and pleased that I was ready to leave the special program, but they also seemed a little concerned that I would now be competing with "regular" kids in Head Start. Head Start is a government-supported preschool for children of low-income families and children with disabilities. They reserved about 10 percent of their registration slots for children with special needs.

I fit in just fine at Head Start. I knew more about raising my hands to take turns than some of the other kids. I had more classroom experience. Remember, I had been going to school for almost three years, since I was about three months old. This was the first time away from home, and in a school setting, for many of my new classmates. The other kids thought that I was extra smart because I had already learned some sign language.

I had learned how to use sign language at a special nonprofit agency called Crippled Children's Society (CCS, now called Via). It was strange: once I learned to say a word, I would stop signing it. My dad was worried that I would get all caught up in signing and stop talking. But the opposite happened-- signing enhanced my desire to speak more. Anyway, the Head Start kids and the kids in our neighborhood thought it was cool that a little kid like me could sign. I felt especially smart and proud of myself. Finally, I could teach the other kids something.

While I was switching to education in the Head Start setting, the speech therapists and the psychologist who had worked with me in Teacher Pat's class continued to see me a couple of times a week in my Head Start classroom. That was a part of my Individual Education Plan (IEP). Public Law 94-142, a federal law passed in 1975, the same year that I was born, guaranteed the education rights of all handicapped children. Finally, we had a legal right to a free, appropriate education, in the least restricted environment. We had a right to go to public schools just like everyone else. Starting at age three, an IEP was a part of the requirements of the law. The IEP listed my learning goals and how I was to reach them. It included therapies that I needed and what transportation would be provided if I needed to be driven to a certain school to better attain my written goals in the plan. This federal law was for kids all over the country, in every state.

Yes, Mom continued to hang around the classroom and help the teacher and other kids just about every day, but she never worked with me. That was okay with me; I knew her job was to help the teacher. We would just smile at each other now and then. If my tongue protruded from my mouth, she would smack her lips together with a very light popping sound, and I would remember that my tongue needed to go back inside. We would smile again at each other. It seemed like keeping my tongue inside of my mouth was just about the hardest thing I had to learn to do at that time of my life. It is amazing, even though I am much older now, Mom can get that smacking sound to work (not that she needs to use it very often anymore, actually almost never).

Head Start was just fine for the next three years. There were field trips to the zoo, picnics in the park, and other great learning experiences. Besides that, Head Start was where I met my first girlfriend; her name was Tia. She had beautiful black skin, big dark brown eyes, curly hair, and a beautiful smile. The most important thing about Tia was, she liked me very much. She would save a seat for me each morning right by her side for singing time, and we would do special projects together during the day. Even though she was called a "regular" kid, and I was a "special " kid, it did not matter to her. I guess she just could not resist such a "handsome dude," as my sister used to call me.

When I was four years of age, I was invited to appear on a television show in San Francisco called *People Are Talking* with host Ross and hostess Ann. My mom wanted everyone to know how much I could do. She was hoping it would raise the expectations others had for children with special needs, including their own parents, the general public, and professionals, especially teachers and physicians. She also wanted the world to know that I was a valuable person, one who was loved by my family, neighbors, and friends.

Whenever I was on television, my parents made sure that I was not wearing clothing that was silky or velvety. Why? Whenever I touched something smooth with my fingers, my tongue seemed to automatically protrude from my mouth. We never knew why that would happen. But we did know why keeping my tongue inside my mouth was harder for me than for most people. It is because my tongue is a bit bigger than average, my muscles are not quite as strong as other people's so they have less control, and most especially, the roof of my mouth is higher than normal. Therefore, my tongue cannot automatically reach its usual resting place when not in use, which is where most tongues go to rest in one's mouth—up on the roof.

In order to get others to have a bit of empathy for my situation, whenever Mom and I would teach a class at a university or at a hospital for doctors, nurses, and social workers, she would ask the participants in the class to stick their tongues out of their mouths. Then she would insist that they keep their tongues out for a very brief amount of time. The students would keep their tongues out for just a few seconds and then retract them. She would then say, "Now you know what a hard job Dean has keeping his tongue in … just as hard as you are having to consciously keep yours out." They would usually all laugh, but I think they got the message. And they learned a valuable old lesson about not judging another person until you have walked a mile in their shoes.

Let us go back to my first television appearance. Mom and I explained all about the different resources, information, laws, and service agencies available to help children with special needs and their families. After that, we shared the importance of connecting families to each other, and the critical need to let families know how they could best find, access, utilize, and even improve systems of care for their children and themselves.

We chatted about the benefits of having mentor parents, who shared their experience of parenting a child with special needs to help other parents; especially new parents, and/or those experiencing a new transition in their child's life. While many different professionals bring to the table great information from their particular areas of expertise, only the parents of children with special needs are the experts on raising a child with special needs; they can bring valuable information to the table about incorporating these children into the fabric of a family and the broader community.

Mom also shared with them about how her organization Parents Helping Parents, Inc. (PHP) was also providing children better informed professionals and more responsive care systems through PHP's trainings for them on: better ways of interacting with families; how to collaborate and better coordinate a child's care; and how to implement the modern concepts of family-centered care being written into new guidelines. One of PHP's most popular trainings was for physicians; it was entitled, "Better Ways of Breaking Diagnostic News." If done poorly, it could damage the bonding between parent and child.

Then the host and hostess of the show turned to me and asked, "Do you have a girlfriend? What is her name?"

I shyly said, "Yeah. Tia."

Boy, was I proud of myself. That was the first of several television shows in which I participated with my family. My sister Jill, my brother Keith, and sometimes one of my good friends would sit in the front row in the audience. I always sat on the stage with Mom. I liked it there.

Years later, when Ross and Ann retired from that show, they were asked what their most memorable show was. You guessed it: we were. I was a star.

Just when I was getting comfortable learning my shapes, colors, numbers, and how to speak a few sentences, Head Start came to an end for me. Graduation day was here, complete with paper caps and gowns, balloons, food, hugs, smiles, and tears. We kids were all happy; I didn't know why some of the families were crying. Those two years went fast. I said "bye-bye" to Tia, not realizing that we would be heading off to different schools, and I would never see her again. I hope she is as happy as I am now, all grown up.

I was now five years old and ready for kindergarten. My parents and the school professionals decided that I should spend a year at a school with a special emphasis on speech; this would better prepare me to succeed in kindergarten the following year. So I attended a special public school with an emphasis on enhancing speech, and I also continued to receive extra speech therapy at CCS. The therapy at CCS was paid for by an agency called Loma Prieto Regional Center.

Loma Prieto (now called San Andreas Regional Center) is a state of California agency that funds various therapies, housing, recreation, and other assistance for individuals with special needs. The regional centers are private nonprofit agencies created by legislation called the Lanterman Act. That act obligates the state of California to ensure the welfare and care of all individuals with developmental disabilities.

Lucky me, I still have a regional center care manager, or case manager, who helps coordinate my services and helps oversee my well-being. They also will pay for respite care if parents feel they need it. The regional center never had to pay for my parents' respite. I am proud to say that Mom and Dad have been lucky; besides me being a great, happy kid, we have a big family of enough aunts, uncles, brothers, sisters, cousins, and friends to spend time with me if Mom and Dad want to go to Reno or Vegas and play the ca-ching, ca-ching machine or if they want to just take off for one of their quarterly "honeymoons." (When I was a little kid, I always wondered what the heck a "quarterly honeymoon" was. I thought that perhaps they paid someone a quarter to get a close look at the moon. Of course, now I know better than that, since I have been on my own honeymoon. Parents can say some of the strangest things when you are a kid.)

For five years, Mom would drive me to school and help in the classrooms or do other volunteer duties around the school while she waited to drive me back home again. One day I heard her telling my dad, "I think I can handle the bus ride now." I thought, "*What? Is she going to ride the bus to school?*" I did not know that what she meant was that *she* could now handle *me* riding the bus; whereas before, she was worried that I might get lost, or sick, or bothered by someone. Now, she felt that I was ready, and so was she.

All the times she had driven me to school, Mom had made a point of telling me to know where the school office was located. She would show me the office and point to the word *Office* on the door. And she encouraged me to ask others where the office was if I could not find it. She let me know that the office was a place where you can get help if you need it. One day, that information came in very handy. The bus driver dropped us off at the wrong school. All the other kids just stood outside the strange school and cried. I looked for the office, found it, went inside, and told the lady at the desk, "Me no here." She asked, "Who are you?" I said, "Dean A. A. Poyadue." She checked some papers, made a phone call, and got all of us kids another bus to our school. She also called my mom and told her that I had "saved the day."

Mom decided that the best way to transition to taking the bus to school was for my first trip to be on the way home (toward a happy and familiar place). So she drove me to school as usual and told me that I would get to ride a little yellow bus back home with my friends. She also showed me the bus and explained how easy it would be to get on and off of it. "Great!" I said. But I quietly thought, "*Okay Mom, I hope this works.*"

The ride home was a little scary, but it was okay. I could see out of the window on the bus; I waved good-bye as the bus driver dropped each of my friends off at his or her home. I was anxiously waiting to see that white house of ours (ours was—and still is—the only white house on the block).

About thirty minutes after we had left my school, I arrived home; Mom was waiting outside to greet me—along with two of our older neighbors, whom I knew as Mr. Joe and Mrs. Lengels (at the time, I thought they must have been a hundred years old; now I know they were only about seventy years of age). They told my mom that if she ever needed someone to meet me at the bus, they would be happy to do it and watch me until she got back—and they did just that several times. They were great neighbors; I remember that they would bring me Halloween candy and then return to their homes and close it down for the night, as they did not want to participate in trick or treating.

I bounded off the bus, ran toward Mom, and gave her legs a big hug. This bus thing *was* going to work out. For a week, Mom drove me to school, and I rode the bus home. Then Mom and I were ready for me to take the bus both ways. The bus picked me up at my house, just like a cab, about 7:15 A.M. every school morning; off we would go to pick up the other students, one by one, and on to our school. At the end of the school day, I eagerly and happily rode the bus home. No problem.

When the month of June arrived, it was time for summer school. I always attended summer school, so I could keep learning and retain the things I had learned by not having big time breaks from school. For some reason, summer sessions were always held at a different school, so I became very used to changes. My sister and brothers would probably have been upset if they had to change schools every year, but not me. They stayed at the same school for eight years. Ugh! How boring. They never went to summer school. I'm sorry for them; it was fun. When Jill went to high school, she decided to take some summer classes. Just like me, she liked it very much and signed up for more summer sessions every year. She was ready for college in three years.

After a year of attending that special speech school and summer school, I was ready to tackle kindergarten. I heard Mom proudly telling her friends that it was a regular kindergarten; I would be pulled out of class for one hour each day to work with a program specialist, a special teacher. That specialist worked with me to help strengthen all my skills—my writing, math, and word recognition; understanding school routines; as well as my speech, physical coordination, and confidence. She was terrific! Thanks to her, I completed kindergarten on schedule, without any major problems.

First grade, look out! Here I come.

Here comes Dean Archibald Anthony Poyadue.

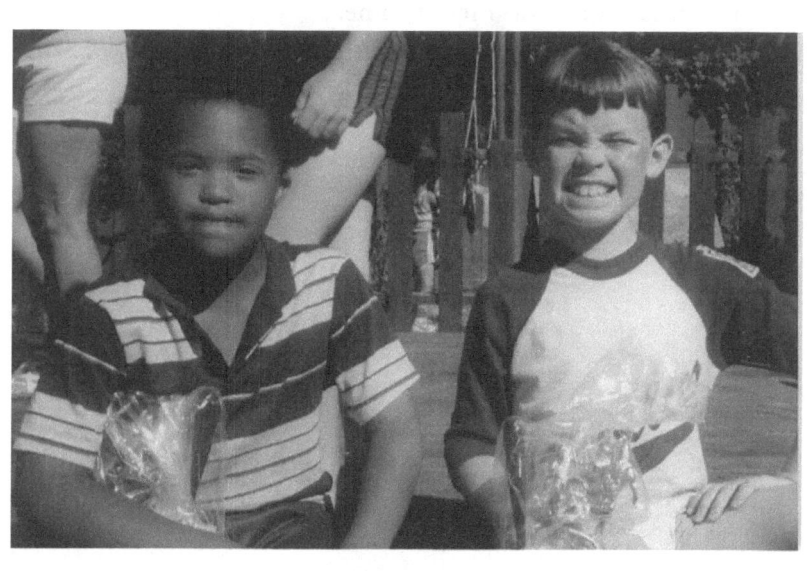

Chapter 2
6–12 Years of Age

Making Progress and Making Friends

Wow! This was new. There was a *man* standing in front of the class. *A male teacher; this is different*, I thought.

I was at Miller Elementary School, the same school as kindergarten, and I kept the same program specialist to help me at least one hour a day. The same little yellow bus brought me to and from my home. My first grade classroom was a short walk from the bus stop. This was going to be easy.

Mom decided to take a few months off from volunteering at my school. Now all I had to do was get use to that man up front. I was settling in well at school at seven years of age.

In January, Mom received a note from my teacher. He said that I was "stuck" on one set of spelling words. On Mom's first visit back to the classroom, she saw that the teacher had written five words on cards about the size of a sheet of paper and hung about twenty of these cards on the classroom wall. The teacher said that I had done well learning to spell all the words on each card until I got to the ninth card. I could spell four of the five words on the card, but I kept misspelling one of the words. Therefore, the teacher would not let me proceed to the other cards until I got that word right.

My mom listened to the teacher and then suggested two ideas. (You know my mom by now; she probably had more ideas but stopped with two.) She said that even though she was basically a good speller, there were still certain words that can trip her up, and she often misspells them. Perhaps this word was one of Dean's "trip-up" words, she said, adding, "It would be a shame to let that one word stop his spelling growth." She asked the teacher, "How about letting him continue with the other word lists and come back to this one later?"

The teacher did not like breaking his rules, but he could see that Mom had her heels dug in, so he let me start the next list of words. She also suggested the following: I needed glasses, so perhaps the location of my seat and the position of the tenth list made it difficult for me to correctly see the words. Could the words be written on a sheet of paper and placed on my desk? "Sure, why not?" the teacher agreed. Mom said it was so nice to be collaborating with the teacher so that they could both help me be successful. Mission accomplished.

I continued to spell most of the words on the other spelling lists. On some lists, I spelled them all correctly, and on others I would misspell one or two, just like my sister and brothers misspelled some words on their spelling lists. Mom wondered why the school demanded 100 percent from me before I could move ahead when they did not demand that of the "regular" kids. Everybody makes a C or D sometimes, but they continue to move forward.

As important as education was, there was more to my life than just school. But the right school, the right education plan, and the right teacher were all extremely important for me, for my ongoing progress, and for my development. Actually, they are very important for every kid, because I hear my brothers and sister talking about how important these same things are for my little nieces and nephews, and they do not have special needs at all. So it seems to me that in order to be successful, all children should start school sooner rather than later. They all need the right programs and smart, caring, dedicated teachers like Teacher Pat, teachers who believe that they can learn.

The school gave me my first IQ test, a nonverbal test. My score was 93. I did not know it at that time, but I later learned that my mom's first IQ score was just 81. She always said that either the IQ test needed revising, or one can do a heck of a lot with 81 (she had graduated salutatorian from her high school class and valedictorian from her nursing school). Everyone was quite pleased with my score; I had no thoughts about it. I just knew that I enjoyed going to school and making friends.

At this same time, I got a chance to go on several "fun" trips. No, not "field" trips, but fun trips. On one such trip, my friend Joey, his mom, and me and my mom flew to Canada. I saw a doctor there. He was friendly, and we got along just fine. He examined me and saw no special health problems; he said I was healthy and growing into a fine big boy.

We stayed in a great hotel, ate fancy foods in the restaurants, and took in the special sites of the city. The next few years, I made similar trips to Las Vegas and San Diego to see doctors who were interested in studying the growth and development of special needs children. People say that travel is one of the best ways to grow in knowledge and ability; I was well on my way to knowing a whole lot and meeting many interesting people along the way. Mom said we were seeing these doctors to help me stay healthy, not to treat me for some kind of illness.

We drove to Las Vegas with another friend from school. That was a long ride, but we stopped and had a picnic along the way. I saw another doctor there, who prescribed some special vitamins for me. They tasted terrible; we had to crush them because I couldn't swallow the pill. We put it in applesauce to help the medicine go down. Even now, as an adult, I still use the good old applesauce routine when I have to take a pill, like Zocor, which keeps my cholesterol number down.

The doctor also gave us homeopathic drops, which were just fine. They had no taste, and I could swallow them easily. The doctor told us that the Queen of England used homeopathic medicines sometimes. I said that my taking the drops meant that I was a "prince" of a guy. My sister agreed.

My parents wanted to include the holistic approach as well as conventional medicine to my health care. Doctors say that more people are doing that now: using acupuncture, acupressure, herbs, lifestyle changes, massage, yoga, and other alternative forms of health care, along with regular traditional care.

Now that I think about it, there was one strange thing about our trips to Las Vegas. Mom likes to play the slots. There we were, in the heart of slot machine country, and she was not playing. Why? I have since learned that she did not start having fun with the slots until after she retired and joined her church's Senior Club. The Senior Club would take field trips to the nearby casinos. Mystery solved.

Going to San Diego was one of our most exciting trips of all. Mom drove to the San Jose airport, and we caught a three o'clock flight to San Diego. When we arrived, we took a cab to the train station.

We boarded the train and headed for a small town outside of San Diego. When we arrived, Mom made a phone call, and a limousine came to pick us up and take us to a doctor's office. After he examined me, we went out to dinner at one of our favorite restaurants. This doctor agreed with the other doctors that I had seen, and we never had to make that trip again.

After dinner, we took the limousine back to the train station, boarded the train for a brief ride, and then took a cab back to the airport. On the way to the airport, I looked out the window of the cab and saw some ships docked in the water. I excitedly asked Mom, "We taking boat today?" Mom laughed and said, "No, Dean, not today, but one day we will. You and I, out to see the world." And take a boat we did: one night we went on the *Hornblower ship* for dinner and dancing in San Francisco.

And my high school graduation gift was a seven-day cruise to Venezuela, Aruba, and other exotic places. (This came after my trip across the good old USA on a train, another special treat with my parents.)

But I've digressed; back to our whirlwind San Diego trip. We landed back in San Jose, and after a brief ride on a bus we picked up our car in the long-term parking lot. Can you believe it? We were home in San Jose by nine o'clock the same evening that we had earlier parked the car in that lot. I smiled and thought, "*What an exciting life I have*".

Yes, we made quite a few trips to see health professionals, but I had only two or three minor health problems. One problem was that I kept spitting up whenever I would drink regular milk. We discovered that I was allergic to milk, so I was started on a soy product. Problem solved, and not just for me.

Mom shared this information with other parents whose kids were spitting up. She would always say, "Tell your doctor about it; maybe it is just an allergy to milk, and all you need to do is change to soy milk. It is certainly worth a try because it is not an expensive thing, it doesn't hurt, and it is not surgery or a major invasive procedure—*just a simple change of milk*. If it doesn't help, the doctor can always keep looking for other answers to the child's problem."

Some kids who are called "special" can have unexpected health or educational problems, which even some professionals may never have experienced. Therefore, families have to become informed and speak up when seeking services that are appropriate for their child's needs. Families should work collaboratively with the dedicated professionals providing services to their child in order to get the best care.

I had three other health problems: my lower jaw was not evenly aligned with my upper jaw, I had one undescended testicle (one testicle was not in the scrotal sac, but had remained inside my body), and I had an inguinal hernia. These might sound like a lot of illnesses, but they were not really bad, did not make me sick, and they did not slow my growth and development. I was actually really healthy; some years, I did not miss even one day of school.

My facial specialist physician said that I should wait until I had finished growing before fixing my jaw—if I wanted to fix it at all. I might be eighteen years of age or older by then. Or, I could live a perfectly normal life without fixing it. Wow! Good! The doctor still saw me once or twice a year just to check on how things were going with my "out-of-line" jaw.

My other doctor thought they should operate on my undescended testicle within the next year or two. When I was eight years old, they surgically moved the testicle from inside my abdomen and put it in my scrotal sac on the outside of my body. How exciting! Now I had a matched pair like my dad and brothers. I came through the surgery with flying colors. Speaking of colors, my hospital room was filled with multicolored balloons, flowers, and candy when I returned from the recovery room. I was back home in a couple of days.

Wow! What a year, and another goal accomplished. To top off the celebration of a successful surgery, my speech therapist, Mrs. J., came to visit and brought me a special gift. I could always count on Mrs. J. for some fun. Speech lessons often included games and outings with her two sons, who were about my age.

The hernia literally cured itself, which sometimes happens after you have that testicle surgery. I was glad no surgery was necessary for the hernia.

After x-rays showed no problems with the bones of my neck, I was cleared to take part in sports. They x-rayed my neck area for cervical spine axial instability. My neck structure was stable and strong enough for playing sports. All kids with Down syndrome who want to play sports should probably have this x-ray done, just to be on the safe side.

Mom signed me up for regular Little League games; she made a special effort to introduce me to the coaches and explained what a "special" player they were going to be privileged to train that season. She let them know how hard I would work for the team and assured them I could understand instructions if they would simply take a little time to not only tell me what I needed to do but also demonstrate new things a couple of times.

Sometimes those demonstrations could be accomplished by just letting me observe the other players take their turn at a new activity, and then I would be good to go. I am what they call a kinesthetic learner. That means I learn best by observing and hands on doing. Auditory learners can just listen to what is being taught and learn it that way; and of course visual learners have got to see it, so they are often reading and writing things down. Heck, a couple of times, I understood the next move before the other kids, who were often horsing around and not paying attention while the coach was showing us how to do something. I would be watching what the coach was doing and listening to his every word. I have a good memory (many people with Down syndrome do, you know), and Teacher Pat had taught me to pay attention when teachers and others are talking.

In addition to baseball, I also tried soccer and basketball. I have to admit that I was no David Beckham when it came to soccer, but it was fun. I was no Michael Jordan either when it came to basketball, but with my excellent eye-hand coordination, I was rather good at putting the ball through the hoop. The basketball coaches were glad to have me on the team. I had a secret weapon at home when it came to basketball: my older brother Keith. He played basketball and became a coach after he graduated from high school. He helped me with sports, while my sister Jill helped me with things like math and spelling.

My mom often tells the story of how she was explaining to Jill that her new baby brother might take a bit longer to learn some things; Jill said, "Oh, that means *slow* learning, not *no* learning; I'll teach him." And that she did. She even set up a little classroom for me with a desk in the corner of our family room. For some strange reason, she called the classroom area "China." Whatever she called it, I was learning reading, writing, and arithmetic. It must run in the family, because Jill's daughter Mira (who is my godchild) insisted that her mom sign her up for a class teaching the Chinese language after kindergarten, and she loved being immersed in Mandarin.

My oldest brother, Turhan, is much older than me. By the time I was born, he had already finished college, found a job, and had an apartment of his own; so he and I did not spend much time together until I began to watch professional wrestling. When the World Wrestling Federation was in town, he took me to see it live, not just on television. What a treat!

Not to be overshadowed by my oldest brother's act of kindness, when Jill finished college, she took me to a Janet Jackson concert (I loved both Michael and Janet Jackson). Then my brother Keith took me to a special Neil Young concert to benefit the Bridge School. The Bridge School is an innovative educational program that was founded by singer Neil Young and his wife Pegi to serve children with special needs. Like I said before, life was great. Dear old sibling rivalry paid off big, with much fun for me.

Besides doing things with my brothers, my sister, and their friends, I did a lot with Pete, my very best friend forever. We made our first communions together, were altar boys together, took family vacations together, went to summer camps together, and we were almost always at special events as a duo, and of course we signed up for the same sports teams. Baseball was his favorite sport. Pete was called a "regular" kid, but my mom said he was anything but regular. She says that he is the most special kid she ever met.

When we were kids, he played first base or catcher, and I played in the outfield or pitched. I did not have a favorite player, but he loved Ricky Henderson. He often read me a book, and I would show him a few basketball moves. We were a balanced pair, helping each other and having fun together; we went to birthday parties, to amusement parks, and raised Peter's 4-H pig together. I don't know if people stared at us because he was a "regular" kid and I was a "special" kid, or because I was black and he was white. You know how some people feel about that black/white thing in

America. All we knew is that we got along well, and we just liked each other.

Pete and I are two old married men now. I am Uncle Dean to Pete's little boy, who is already a lot like his dad, because he and I get along just fine. Pete is an attorney; of course, he and I are still best friends and stay in touch. Oops! There I go, jumping ahead again. Sorry.

Back to sports when I was younger. I had a strong throwing arm and was a better baseball pitcher than the opposing team ever expected. I also had good eye-hand coordination (even though I flunked my first major eye-hand coordination test at school; I'll tell you about that later). Anyway, the other team's players were so surprised by my throwing ability that they often swung the bat and completely missed the ball. My coach called me his "secret weapon." Our team more often won the game than loss. I was getting bigger, and sports and music were starting to be a lot of fun.

One day, Mrs. J., my speech therapist, called my mom at her office. "When you come to pick up Dean," she said, "stop in and talk awhile; we have a bit of a problem." My mom wondered what the problem could be. Was my hesitating speech worsening? Did I say something inappropriate? Did I do something inappropriate?

Mom had prepared herself for negative news from Mrs. J., as that was often the case when a professional wanted to talk to you about your child. She could remember only one time that she had received a phone call with good news from a professional working with me. When I was in sixth grade, the school tester called her to say I had done a wonderful job during the testing period. She said that I had stayed focused and did not tire before the tests were completed, and she complimented me for showing her I knew about how to operate the computer.

Before we get back to Mrs. J.'s call, another tester had called to tell Mom I had flunked my eye-hand coordination test. Mom had to keep herself from laughing. Instead, she asked, "What did you use to test him?"

The tester answered, "We have them put beads on a string. They have to put at least five beads on the string to get a score."

Mom asked, "Couldn't Dean put a bead on the string?"

"Oh yes," the tester answered, "but he only put on one. And we can't tell them that they need to do more."

At this point, my mom chuckled and said, "Dean does not like to do repetitive behaviors. I am sure he was thinking, 'There, I've done that; what's next?'"

Mom went on, "Let me tell you some things he can do, and you let me know if these things are examples of good eye-hand coordination. He often gets four out of five shots at the free throw line in basketball; he can pitch a baseball across the plate in the strike zone quite often. And he not only beats me, but most of his older brother's friends when they come over to play bumper pool."

The tester agreed that if I could do those things, I did indeed have very good eye-hand coordination. Issue settled.

Mom explained to the tester that this is why it is so important for parents, teachers, and health professionals to discuss things, listen to each other, and share the information that they each know about the child in order to solve problems and prevent misdiagnosis or wrong evaluations, which can lead to misguided approaches to education or health care interventions. And now, back to Mrs. J.'s dilemma.

Mom came into Mrs. J's home, where I had finished my speech therapy for the week. Mrs. J. explained, "I gave Dean a homework assignment: He was to cut some pictures from a magazine, and we would use them for our speech discussion. All of the pictures are rather naughty, shall we say."

Mom looked at my collection of pictures and breathed a sigh of relief. I had used pictures from my brother's *Playboy* magazine to complete the assignment. Mom reassured Mrs. J. that all was well.

"He *is* a growing boy," Mom said, "and boys like to look at

Playboy pictures. I'll give him some different magazines tonight to redo the assignment."

Mom continued, "I am so glad you brought this to my attention; I will talk to his older brother about keeping his stuff out of the reach of the younger children. And don't hesitate to call my office or home if you have any other concerns. Besides, it is always good to chat with you. See you next week."

I really wasn't worried about the pictures. Being a nurse, Mom is used to naked bodies and things. Whenever she was going to give me a shot, or check me for some sickness, I would say to her, "Mom, you turning into a nurse now?" I think it is a good idea to let people know when you are "changing hats"—going from mom to nurse, or from friend to teacher, from parent to professional, and so on. Everyone in our family was always showing Mom some part of their body to see if it was swollen, or red, or not looking right.

Even the neighbors used to show her parts of their bodies if they were not feeling too good. In our family, we also talked about all the parts of the body and how they worked. And we tried to learn and use the correct names for the body parts and functions. I remember one day, a young neighbor boy was visiting, and he was squirming around a lot. Jill asked him, "Do you have to urinate?" He said, "I don't speak French, but I got to pee-pee."

Jill also informed Mom that the other kids told us that we had it wrong when we talked about having a "bowel movement." They said the word is *poop, do-do,* or *caca.* My parents assured us that all these words were perfectly okay. They said that different people in different cultures, different areas, and different countries all use different words-- all okay.

Besides those rather humorous incidents concerning our anatomy and physiology (we never called any of it sex education— perhaps schools should switch), there were a few other incidents that probably turned Mom's hair a little gray, including the following stories (I must have been a pretty good kid, cause her hair is still plenty black these days, even past her seventy-sixth birthday).

The scariest thing that happened to me was being left on the school bus. The bus driver had picked me up, as usual, at about 7:15 A.M., and he picked up the other kids that rode the bus to my school. As the story was told to Mom, he dropped them all off at school but did not realize that I was asleep in my seat. After parking the bus for some time, he realized that I was still on there. He drove me to my school and let me out of the bus on the street corner; he did not even help me get to my classroom or explain to my teacher what had happened. Mom was livid when the school called her to let her know about the incident. For months she drove me to school and picked me up the remainder of the school year.

When I was near the end of first grade, Mom visited the second grade classroom to meet the teacher. She was thrilled with the teacher's methods of inclusion and her techniques for working with children with special needs. So during my IEP planning session, everyone agreed that I would be in that teacher's classroom next school year. It would be perfect for me. When school started, I was assigned to that room. But in less than four weeks, I was out of there.

The teacher *was* perfect, but her aide was an awful, controlling, ego-crushing, confidence-shattering drill sergeant. She would not let me do things that I had learned the year before, such as getting my own coat or finding my way to the bus stop. She did not want us kids to make a move without her involvement. Mom thought I might lose confidence in my ability to make even simple choices if I remained in that classroom setting. A transfer to a different classroom was in order. Decisions are not set in concrete, even well developed ones, if they turn out to have a negative effect on the child. Lucky for me --a great teacher and a wonderful aide awaited me at another school where I learned a lot. They continued to nurture my independence, and I grew in knowledge and self-assurance. I think that was probably the beginning of my transition to independent living.

Near the end of second grade, we created a new IEP for the next school year. My third grade year would be at yet a different school, with Mr. Barrett. As I said before, change was not a problem for me. I expected new schools every fall and every summer. I found some really good friends at this new school; I loved recess, when I had the greatest time playing with my friends Paulo and John.

Mom was a bit unnerved when she visited my new school and found me climbing the tall backstop on the baseball field, as two yard monitors were deep in conversation (instead of paying attention to what was going on with the kids). At so many schools, it seems that at the beginning of the school day, at recess, and immediately after school ends, there is a need for more adult supervision. There was often too much rough play; bullies often had a field day, timid kids were lonely and isolated, and kids like me tried new things that were unsafe.

Believe it or not, we returned to the same school for fourth grade. We headed straight for the same classroom that I had been in the previous year. I entered the classroom but quickly moved backward to leave.

Mom said, "What's the matter?"

I said, "I've done Barrett." (Mr. Barrett, my third grade teacher, had given me permission to call him just Barrett, because I had trouble saying the word *Mister*.)

Mom said, "I know you had Mr. Barrett last year; he is going to teach fourth grade this year, so you will have him again."

"Oh, okay," I said, "Barrett and I get along just fine." I did not mind staying at this same school, because my good friends were still in this class.

About this time in my life, Mom and I often watched a television show called *Life Goes On*. The main character's name was Corky Riley. One day, I said to my mom, "Corky has Down syndrome."

Mom said, "Yes, he does."

I asked, "I have Down syndrome?" I thought that Corky kind of looked like me.

Mom said, "Yes, you do."

I laughed out loud and said, "No, Mom, I *used* to have it, but not anymore."

Mom said, "Downs is not something that goes away, but if you feel like no Downs today, who am I to rain on your parade?" That was the end of the topic … for the time being.

Speaking of parades, I had won a United Way art contest for special kids. The local United Way was celebrating twenty-five years of service to the community. I thought it would be a great idea to just write all the numbers from 1 to 25 and frame them. Believe it or not, I won first place and was in the lead car of the Thanksgiving Day parade, which ushered in Santa's visit to town. It was great fun!

A few months after our conversation about Corky Riley and Down syndrome, Mom and I were driving to my music therapy lesson. I was learning how to play the piano and the violin. My sister was taking piano lessons, so I wanted to do that. And my best friend, Pete, was taking violin lessons, so I wanted to do that too.

In a matter-of-fact manner, I casually said to Mom, "I have Downs like Corky."

Just as casually, she replied, "Yup." And we immediately went on to another topic, talking about our plans after my piano and violin lessons. I think she realized that I had finally gotten it: that thing about "no cure," and being something that is not "going away" that I talked about earlier. I was about twelve years old, and I got it.

So we went on to my music therapy, as I added, "It will be great to stop by the bakery and have a donut on the way back home." And so we did.

By the way, Mom told me that I probably had an easier time with math because of the many music lessons I had taken. One of my music classes was actually taught by a music therapist, and I also had piano lessons with a regular piano teacher. Zenia, a high school student, who could not only play the piano well enough to win contests, but she was also a very good teacher. She often put on little recitals to showcase her students, including Jill and me. Zenia's mother always prepared many good things to eat and drink after the recitals. Although my piano playing was not perfect, no one denied that I did indeed make a most perfect bow after my performance. A few years later, I tried trumpet lessons. Thank God my parents only rented the trumpet, because I did not stick with those lessons very long. Still, I thought the title of Corky's show was right: life does indeed go on, and life is good.

In addition to all of my schooling, and speech and music therapy, about twice a year I saw a therapist from the Human Potential Program, based in Philadelphia. He would come to San Jose, look me over, and give Mom some suggestions of how to boost my potential in many areas. He prescribed certain activities that I needed to do several times a week.

I remember us having family meetings once a week to decide what household chores everyone would be responsible for in the coming week. Besides deciding who would do the dishes, take out garbage, and pick things up, one of the jobs involved the four boxes that contained things to "boost my potential." My parents could then post the schedule, and we could do our jobs without having to be told or constantly reminded. We all liked that approach.

Mom, Dad, Jill, and Keith would rotate who did which box with me for the coming week. They would work (or play, as it seemed to me) with the items in the boxes at least once each day for 15 to 30 minutes. For example, one box contained a small handheld vibrator, a soft mitt, and some cotton. Whoever had that box would rub my skin with the various things in the box to stimulate my sensitivity and awareness. Another box contained small jars of vanilla, cinnamon, and wonderfully smelling perfume. I would briefly smell each one to stimulate my sense of smell. I did not have to know the names of the items, but it wasn't long before I could call them by name.

Another box contained pictures of animals, household items, and other objects; whoever was working with this box would show me a picture and name the item. By flashing the cards quickly, that kept me interested, and I learned many things that way. One box held cards that boosted my math skills. Each card had dots that took the shape of a different number. For example, the five dots on the number five card were arranged in the shape of the number 5. My family member would simply flash the card and say the word *five*.

One of the best things about these boxes was that my family was not supposed to test me. No testing meant less resistance on my part; we just worked (played) with the materials in the boxes and had fun for at least twenty minutes a day. My parents believed that this targeted stimulation also added to my ability to successfully handle math and spelling later in junior high.

Keith always liked getting what they called "the gross motor box"; he and I would take a walk, run, climb a ladder, or hang on the monkey bars. He especially liked the spinning exercise. He would sit me on a table or in a chair that he could rotate, first one way and then the other. Sometimes he would hold me in his arms and swing me around. This helped my balance and muscle strength, but I think my brother just enjoyed making me get dizzy. Whether for dizzy or duty, I knew we would have a real fun time. My sister Jill preferred the flash cards with math and words and pictures, so she and Keith would often swap boxes if they happened to choose the one they liked the least.

There was much more to that development game, but you get the idea. It was fun, and we all loved being together as a family. Family meetings each week were also fun. We took turns being in charge; we each got to choose where to hold the meeting (in the family room, on the sun porch or elsewhere), what food or drinks were served, and what topics would be discussed we put on the agenda.

There was always learning going on in my life. But not just in my life, my sister's and brother's also. Mom used to say, "It's what you do with what you got; it doesn't matter how much you got." She would add, "You can be endowed with a lot, but if you do nothing with it, that is much worse than having partial potential and using it to the max to make a successful life for yourself."

And she would end with, "What's our motto, Dean?"

And I would say, "Can do; if I can't, I try."

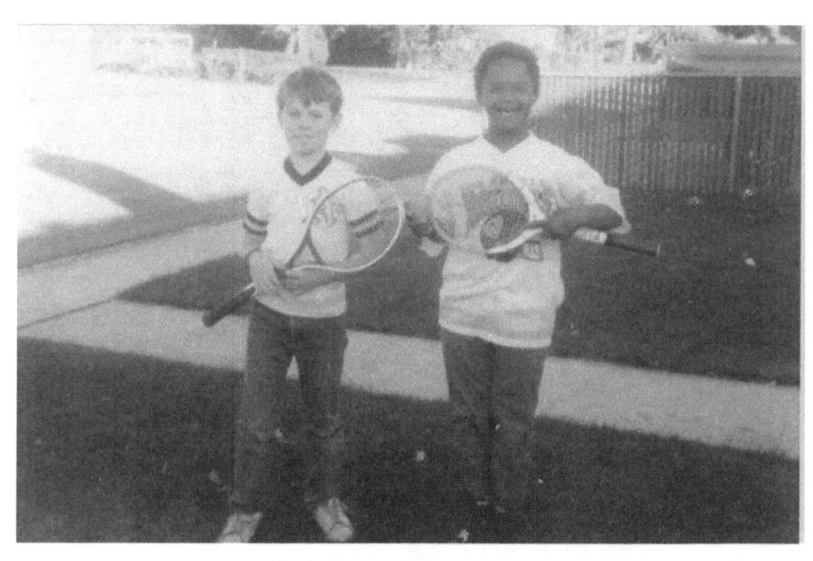

Chapter 3
12–15 Years of Age

Moving On and Up

Our main education goal in fifth grade was preparing me for junior high (grades six, seven, and eight). Many parents dreaded the junior high school campus as opposed to an elementary school setting, and my mom was no exception.

As a part of the preparation for junior high, we decided that I should definitely try to master cursive writing. When Mom brought it up, the teacher balked, and Mom did not argue. Boy, was I surprised. She did not try to convince the teacher at all. I guess that she chose what she wanted to fight about, and this was not one of the times she chose to fight.

Another lesson learned: choose your battles; there is usually not enough energy or time to fight them all. Later that day, we visited Ann, Mom's friend (and my friend Pete's mother). Ann was a great teacher; she even taught swimming to most of the kids in the neighborhood, including me and my brother and sister.

Ann was busy raising her family at this time, so she only did substitute teaching for the schools when she could. Most of the time, she did after school care for a lot of her friends. Mom asked her to introduce cursive concepts to me on Fridays. I loved waiting there for Mom to pick me up on Fridays, because Pete and I could play. Ann agreed to take on the job, and it was not long before everyone took great pride in saying to me, "Write your name in cursive." I would say, "Sure, why not?" That was my favorite answer, not only to that request, but also to many others: "Sure, why not?"

My friendship with Pete grew as we grew. We continued to do many things together. He was that "regular" kid and I was that "special" kid. But you remember what my mom always said (and she still does): "Peter is the most special kid I ever met." Why, just thinking about our wonderful relationship can almost bring her to tears of joy. As we matured, he and I continued to be on the same sports teams, we took swimming lessons together, and periodically visited Disneyland and Great America, and showed Pete's pig at the county fair.

One summer, Pete went with us for a vacation to San Diego. It was strange how sometimes the hotel clerks would direct their comments and questions to Pete instead of my mom and dad. My parents would let the clerk know that Pete was with us, and they were in charge of arrangements. Mom thought the confusion might be because we were black and Pete was white; maybe they thought that he was not with us. We could not figure out why people might be staring, and we were having too much fun to care or waste our time on that.

The Wild Animal Park in San Diego was the best. The people visiting the park were put in cages that moved about, and the animals were free to roam wherever they pleased. This was just the opposite of most parks we had visited, where the animals were in cages and the people were free to roam about, staring at them.

You will hear more about Pete and me later. But I must admit right here and now that Pete was always better than me at talking and reading, and I could always beat him at bumper pool and basketball. Our birthday parties were always a blast for both of us. We were like "the brain and the brawn." We were an unbeatable duo.

This was a really good time of my life. I know that about now you must be thinking that life was always just "really good" for me. But no, there were a few bad days, and I will share one or two with you … later.

Pete and I also went off to summer camp at Santa Clara University. We spent a week in the dorms there. As my luck would have it, our room was right across from the swimming pool … pretty college girls in bikinis were lounging by the pool all day. During the morning hours, we played many different sports, other types of games, and hobbies. In the evening, we participated in social activities and had contests. Guess who won the dancing contest? Yes sir, me. It was so much fun! Besides dancing, I gained a lot of confidence in my ability to do many other things during camp that week, like finding my way from one place to the other and making my needs known to the camp counselors. Boy, I hated to see that week come to an end.

About a week after returning home, I asked my brother Keith to take me to Pete's house so I could swim. He said sure, so off we went. As he settled back in a lounge chair to watch me, I walked to the edge of the diving board and proceeded to dive in. Keith almost had a heart attack, because before going to camp I would hardly put my face under the water during swimming lessons with Pete's mom. My brother was ready to dive in and get me when I surfaced and swam to the other side of the pool. After his heart stopped racing, he couldn't wait to get home and share the exciting news with the rest of the family. He couldn't stop saying, "Dean can swim and dive." I sure could, and I enjoyed it.

Summer was over all too soon, and I was off to junior high. My teacher was Ms. Turner, an award-winning teacher. Really, she did win an award for her great teaching expertise, and I think it must have been for caring for us students as well. She was good at letting us know that she believed that we could learn. And I loved how she would always eliminate about ten of the twenty problems on our math homework paper; she would say, "If you can do those ten, I know you can do the other ten; so do a good job with just those ten problems."

I thought Ms. Turner had really gone a bit too far when she gave me fractions to work with. I got up enough courage and told her, "Ms. Turner, this is hard for me."

She said, "I know, Dean, but remember when I gave you long division and you thought it was hard, and it was, but remember, you did it."

She really had a way of getting me to try things that I was unfamiliar with and getting the best out of me. Yes, I started to understand fractions (adding and reducing fractions, and finding least common denominators) and spelling words like "Thanksgiving" and "grandmother." I was on a roll again. I could not wait to get home and do my homework every evening. I would not let Mom and Dad go to bed until I had finished all my work, because I knew Ms. Turner would be waiting for me to hand it in the next day. She would smile at me and say, "Dean, your homework please." And I would proudly pull it out and place it neatly on her desk.

I was doing so well I was able to take on a job at school. At the appropriate time, I would go to the office, pick up the mail, and distribute it to the teachers before returning to my classroom. I was chosen student of the month for the whole school. I received a sticker that my parents proudly displayed on our car's rear bumper.

Now I know that this is going to sound unreal. Mr. Harris, the principal of my elementary school, was transferred to my junior high school the same year I started there. I was really glad that he was there, because I liked him very much.

One day, for some reason, I told my mom that I did not feel like going to school. "Are you sick?" she asked. "Let me feel your head; do you have pain somewhere?" Mom was quickly asking questions and checking me over.

I shook my head no and then said, "I just don't feel like going to school today." This was very unusual for me. I had received awards for perfect attendance for whole school years. I said to Mom, "Let's just go in and talk to Mr. Harris." She agreed.

We went to the school and headed to Mr. Harris's office. He greeted us warmly with a smile and said, "What can I do for you, Dr. Dean?" The kids had started to call me "Dr. Dean" in reference to a television commentator with that name. I said that I just didn't feel like school today.

Mr. Harris asked me some questions about how things were going at school, in the classroom, and on the play yard; were there any new kids giving trouble; and so on. I answered all in the negative. Mr. Harris finally said, "Dean, I can see from your record that so far, you have not missed any school days this year. I think you are absolutely correct; you just need a day off from school. Sometimes, as grown-ups, we just need a day off from work. That is kind of what vacations are all about. I will write a note for you to give to your teacher, letting her know that I am authorizing a day off for you today."

I smiled my favorite wide grin and said, "Thank you, Mr. Harris."

He said, "See you around, buddy."

We left the principal's office and headed for my classroom. I gave the note to Ms. Turner, left school, and had a fun day with my mom at her office. That day, I was probably the only kid in this country who had asked to "go to the principal's office."

I did not miss another day of school that entire semester; even when I hurt my arm so badly playing basketball during recess that I had to go to the doctor; I had to take antibiotics to keep it from getting infected. I still have a scar on my elbow from that bad accident.

Before the school year ended, a lovely lady from Russia came to visit our classroom. She was amazed that children with special needs were actually being taught in regular public schools; she was also surprised that we had laws that guaranteed the rights of all children, including those with disabilities. It was nice having a visitor from a foreign country, especially one as pleasant as this lady.

She often smiled as she asked questions about our room and our school. Because Mom had encouraged her to visit my classroom, there was a story about her visit, and about my education, in the major local newspaper. There were great pictures of me working in the classroom as well. One showed me doing a math problem on the blackboard. I thought, *"There must be special kids all over the world. How neat."*

So the sixth grade came and went. What a wonderful year. The next year, I stayed in Ms. Turner's classroom. Unfortunately for her and me, halfway through the school year, she fell and hurt her leg. We had to have a substitute teacher.

Mom knew something was wrong when she had to start prodding me to do my homework. I told her that the new teacher didn't ask for our homework and did not say anything to us if we didn't turn it in. I was also coming home with less work to do. Mom went in to talk to the teacher. The substitute said she believed that 'we kids' should not be doing fractions and that type of math, and a lot of other things. She also said she was teaching us to be responsible by not asking us for our homework. Mom told her that I was getting the message that she didn't care and that the homework must not be very important. She told her that the students were used to Ms. Turner asking for their homework, and that most of them had become very responsible about doing the work and putting it on her desk.

Mom showed her past math homework papers that I had completed, but to no avail. We were fighting a losing battle. This new substitute teacher would not budge from her two positions: these special needs kids could not learn above the level *she* had set for them, and she was teaching responsibility by not showing any interest in their homework. Although I continued to go to school, most of my progress that year occurred with home learning from my family.

About this time, my friend Pete and I decided to be altar boys at St. John Vianney's Catholic Church. Several years before, we had made our First Communion there. That was another day of celebration and a small mishap. We had to carry lighted candles as we walked from the rear to the front pews of the church. I was so excited that I held my candle a little too close to the girl in front of me. Someone sitting along the aisle saved the day by grabbing my arm to prevent me from walking too close, and adding just a little more space between us. We were all dressed up and had a big party with family and friends when the ceremony was completed. Now we were old enough to be altar servers (they used to call them altar boys, but of course they now let girls do the job also, so we say altar servers).

After a few weeks of practice, Pete and I were ready to don our robes and do our thing. Whenever I was not quite sure about what I should do next, I always moved very slowly, and I would look at the priest's face to see if there was a little smile or a little frown. Mom said that she learned from me as she watched me successfully help the priests during the regular mass services, and I even helped on some special occasions with incense and other things.

She said she learned that when you are in an unfamiliar situation, it is wise to move more slowly (whether walking, talking, or driving a car), and you will be less likely to get into big trouble. Also, observing the reactions of others around you can help you to know how to proceed with whatever you are doing. By the way, when Jill asked to be an altar server, she was told "no" because at that time, it was only for boys to do. Sometimes, I think she is still a little angry at the church about that. She was always very good at just about everything she tried, and I know she would have been great at that job too. That made me a little sad for her.

A new school year arrived. Ms. Turner was back for eighth grade—hooray! We needed to prepare for high school. Things got a little confusing to me because Ms. Turner had had a baby. My mom had often talked about people as either parents or professionals. Now Ms. Turner had turned into a parent. Was she still a professional? The answer I got was, "Yes, professionals can be parents and parents can be professionals."

Mom said now that Ms. Turner is a parent, she will probably

an even better teacher, because she could add her experience as a parent to her teaching abilities. Another lesson learned: parents could also learn a profession, add it to their expertise and enhance their abilities as parents. I learned that people could indeed wear two hats. But, it is easier to wear each other's hats than it is to walk in each other's shoes.

This wearing two hats was just like Pete, who was a "regular" kid, but my mom said he was the most "special" kid she knew. So regular kids can also be special and special kids can be regular at times. I was glad that I was getting this all straightened out before I got to high school. I was beginning to think that maybe we should stop trying to label people and just call Pete, Pete; call Ms. Turner, Ms. Turner; and just call me Dean.

That year, I also realized one of the main reasons "I am special is because I like myself, and I have a family that loves me." I put those exact words on a poster we had to make about ourselves as a class project. Mom thought what I wrote on the poster was important enough to share at a national conference where she gave a speech.

Near the end of the school year, my planning team (my teacher, parents, school psychologist, and others) gathered around a table at school to work on my IEP for next year, for high school. One of the members of the team told Mom that she did not think I could handle a regular high school; she did not agree with those goals and objectives. Mom told her that she would sign a statement that it was her own insistence that we give a regular high school a try, with some regular classes and some special classes.

Mom also encouraged her to write on the IEP that professionally, she thought these goals were too lofty. That way, she would have documentation of her views that could support her if we needed to go to fair hearing or court. Others would know that she was not responsible for the goals written. She agreed to that, and we finished writing my Individual Education Plan.

Our eighth grade graduation ceremony was terrific. It was actually held in the gymnasium of the high school that I would attend the next school year. We had a big party at my house. Lots of friends and family members attended, and of course Teacher Pat was there to congratulate me, along with my four great old aunts: Margaret, Billie, Edna, and Evelyn. Pete and I had our pictures taken together in our graduation gowns since we both were graduating that same day, although he was graduating from a different school. We were both very proud of ourselves.

I had not only survived, I had grown, I had matured, and I had conquered junior high. And for once in my life, there would be no summer session. I was ready for high school.

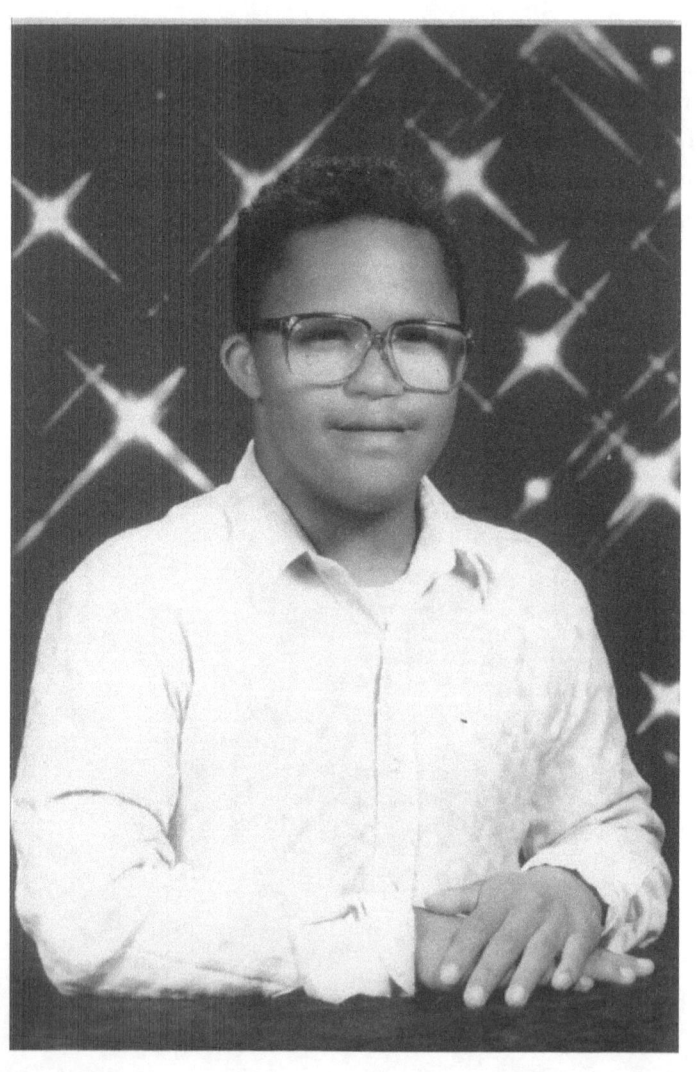

Chapter 4
15–19 Years of Age

High Times

"**N**o, not today Mom! This is high school. I go by myself," I protested.

"But the school is bigger; you have to find your schedule and go to different areas of the campus for your classes. It is not all in one classroom," she said with a voice that held a combination of fear and reassurance.

My big brother Keith said, "One of the kids I coached last year is going to swing by and pick him up, Mom. He's a sophomore at Dean's school. He will drive him to school and help him navigate this first day." Keith continued, "You know this kid. His name is Chris. You and his mom have done some projects together. They live a few miles up the road from us."

For the next three years, Chris picked me up and drove me to school in his car. Mom never had to take me to high school. It was great being with the big man on campus and a football hero, as I strolled across the high school grounds and headed off to class each day.

Chris not only got me to school that first day, but he made sure I found my schedule and showed me to my first classroom. He also came back and pointed me in the right direction to my next class. I am good with directions, so Chris only had to show me that first day, and only once for each class, and then I was good to go. Besides, I was not the only freshman a little scared that day, but I was the only one with a personal escort to help me get started. Boy, was I lucky.

Chris was another one of those "regular" kids that my mom labeled as "very special." He grew up to be an occupational therapist (OT). Wouldn't you know—he chose a helping profession for his life's work. He is still helping people who need a little extra attention and encouragement.

Not only does life "go on," it all seems to "go around and around" and become connected. For example, Dana, my brother Keith's beautiful wife, another really nice person, is an OT also. And wouldn't you know it, Chris was lucky enough to have her as one of his trainers when he was studying in the hospital. Chris helped me; she helped him, and I am sure that some day, someone we know will help her when she needs it, and my turn to help someone will come also. I sure hope so.

I like the idea of everybody helping everybody when they need it, so anyone can make it on their own if they choose to. Mom calls that "interdependence," which she much prefers over the term "living independently".

By the way, Mom continued to come visit my classes once or twice a year, even in high school. She visited both my regular and special classes. I was about a fifty-fifty student: I spent a little more than half of my time in special classes and the rest in regular classes. My favorite regular classes were computer science, photography, art, Spanish, summer math, physical education, and general science. I learned a little Spanish in grade school; it was easier for me to say *"uno, dos, tres"* than *"one, two three."*

I have to admit, speaking fast and clearly was not my strong suit. But whenever Mom asked teachers, students, employers, co-workers, and others about understanding me, they would say they had no trouble understanding me. She finally came to the conclusion that I did not talk a lot, but I communicated well (unlike some people who talk a lot but communicate very little).

I remember the first week of my art class. My teacher, Mrs. O., called my mom and asked her to please come in. Mrs. O. explained to Mom that this was a regular art class; she was not sure whether I was up to it. Mom could not come in right away because she had to go out of town to make a speech. I think mom wanted to give Mrs. O. a chance to work with me and get to know my abilities before she came in. She also wanted me to give the class a chance before deciding whether I could or could not do it.

About two weeks later, Mom came to my class and sat quietly in a corner to see how I was fitting in. Then a strange thing happened as the teacher dismissed the students and started to talk with mom. Mrs. O's first words were, "I can't think of why I called you to come in; Dean is doing just fine. As you can see, he follows my instructions better than many of my other students because he is serious and pays attention." Even if you are not the smartest kid in class, if you are serious, do the work, pay attention, and study, you can still learn a lot and be successful in school.

I think I almost drove the photography teacher out of his mind. My mom's phone must have been ringing a lot that year, as he also called her to come in. He explained how one step in the process of developing the photos needed to be done in a completely darkened room, but I kept turning on the light so I could see what I was doing. Mom had no answer. She simply begged his patience on that issue and asked for some attention to the things I was doing correctly; perhaps those things would get me through. I'm afraid I got a D in that class.

I loved that class though, because we were given special passes to take our cameras around the school campus while everyone else was in their classrooms. I liked learning about using the camera and soon talked my parents into getting me a video camera (later when I was getting ready to go off to college, this was one of the first things I packed). Mom even hired me to video some of her training sessions with other parents and professionals. I must tell you that the pay was very poor. At our house, we were always encouraged to "volunteer" to do things or help someone. And of course, that meant work, but no pay (in money, anyway). Oftentimes, it was a great experience, and I met very interesting people. No money, but I learned a lot.

School was not all work; in my junior year, I got a part-time job at a department store, and more important than that, I had a girlfriend. I think my family thought the "girlfriend" was imaginary, and they were a bit shocked when she came over to our table at the Family Valentine Social to ask me for a dance. Dancing was one of my strong suits when it came to the ladies. At more than one social affair, girls would come over and ask me for a dance, especially after they had a chance to watch me on the dance floor.

One time at a formal dance, I met Kristi Yamaguchi, the famous Olympic ice skater. I also met lots of famous football players that night, like Kena Turner, Ronnie Lott, and Jim Plunkett, who had attended my high school. Ed Rutkoski, a former player for the Washington Redskins, took me around and introduced me to many of his friends and fellow football heroes. They all gave me their autographs on a football that Ed had bought for me. Of course I still have it. The very famous coach, John Madden, was there and gave a speech, but I did not get his autograph; that was my choice, because I am a San Francisco 49er fan all the way, and he used to coach the Oakland Raiders.

By the way, Ed Rutkoski was a really good guy, very caring and very funny. He was always doing something for someone in need. We often helped him sell food and drinks at the NFL Alumni food booth at Candlestick Park before 49er games. Then Ed would make sure we all had good seats when the game started. Ed also made sure some of the profits from the food went to children's organizations, like Parents Helping Parents. At one game, Ed pulled some strings and we got onto the playing field as part of the halftime celebration in honor of children with special needs. I was so sorry to hear that Ed died a few years ago. I had just seen him about a year before that, and as usual, he was making sure everyone was having a good time and laughing. Ed was one of the very "good guys," as my dad would say.

During this time of my life, I often spent Saturday mornings playing tennis at my high school or at a nearby junior college. One Saturday was much more exciting than others: after we finished playing tennis and headed for the parking lot to get our car and return home, Mom got into the car on the *passenger* side. She said, with a sly smile on her face, "You have been wanting to learn to drive; the parking lot is almost empty. Why not start today?"

I didn't say anything; I just hopped into the driver's seat right away before she could change her mind. I couldn't believe it. Was this really happening? I took a deep breath. *Stay cool and calm*, I told myself. She gave me the keys and said, "Before we start, I want to emphasize that there are *two* pedals on the floor of the car. I want to be sure you know what each is for and how to use it. One is for the gas, to make us go, and the other is the brake, to make us stop. Let's practice by moving your foot back and forth from the gas to the brake. Go—stop—go—stop—go—stop."

I did that several times before putting the key in to start up the car. "There is one other little detail you need to be aware of," Mom said. "When you turn the steering wheel, even though you might want to turn the car a lot, you only need to turn the wheel a little."

I said, "Okay."

Mom continued, "You are going to go slowly by just pressing *very lightly* on the gas. You will stop the car by pressing firmly on the brake. And you will turn the wheel very, very, very small amounts to make the car maintain your position in your lane, or to change its position on the road. Are you ready?"

Boy, was I ready! I put the key in the ignition and started the car. I gave it a little gas and was on my way across the parking lot, a bit jerky, of course. But wow! I can't tell you how exciting it was and how grown-up I felt. We spent about thirty minutes on my first driving lesson: twenty minutes talking and ten minutes driving.

Mom congratulated me and said that I had done about as well as my sister and brothers when she taught them.

I can handle a car pretty well. But I do not have a driver's license. It is not the handling of the car, but the handling of all that traffic that I cannot do well. Still, I will never forget that first lesson and other times practicing driving—in the safe environment of an empty parking lot.

I also learned that my mom had let my grandmother take the wheel of her car in an empty parking lot when Grandma was about seventy-five years old; she had never driven a car before. Grandma was a happy camper the day she took the wheel for her first (and last) driving experience. It seems that little things really can mean a lot, to a lot of people. Grandma never forgot it. And neither have I.

The singer Carrie Underwood encourages Jesus to "take the wheel," and I'll bet that there are a lot of regular folks who will never get a license to drive but would get a big kick out of taking the wheel, at least once in their life. I heard that Stevie Wonder and Ray Charles (two guys who are blind) even gave it a try.

I remember one time the mother of a new baby with special needs asked me whether her child would be able to catch a ball or do some other activities. I said, "Our family motto is 'Can do.'"

She asked, "But what if you can't?"

I smiled and said, "At least I try." And I proudly looked at Mom as if I had won the national spelling bee. I like to try, and I think most people like to at least be given the chance to try different things.

On Saturdays we did not go to the tennis court, we were in the bowling alley perfecting my hook. That crazy thing called eye-hand coordination came in handy again. I could often make three strikes in a row. It was great having my own ball and my own shoes, as my interest in bowling grew and continues to this day.

One day after walking home from high school, I tried to open the front door but it would not open. For some reason, it was locked (don't tell anyone, but we never locked the front door back then; of course, we lock it now). I went to the back of the house

48

and started to crawl through one of the windows of our sunroom. I got halfway through, but then I got stuck. Unfortunately, I ended up breaking the glass, but I made it into the house. It was such a funny story, my parents did not even think about punishing me for breaking the window. They said, "At least you were problem solving, and not screaming or crying and making a scene."

I did believe in problem solving. I think it came from our family motto, "Can do, or at least try." For example, Dad, Mom, and I used to take a walk very early in the morning. As we headed toward the hills, we crossed one street that had a signal light. Because it was so early, there was almost no traffic; Dad would look both ways and then cross the street, even if the light was red. That really bothered me. I begged him not to do that, saying, "Please wait for the Walk sign!" But I had no success in stopping Dad's action.

After a few mornings of that, I decided to jog ahead of Dad when we got near that area, and I pushed the crossing button so the "Walk" sign would be on by the time Dad arrived at the corner. Mom said that she was proud of the fact that I had found a solution instead of spending all my time arguing about the problem. She said that was something she learned from me that day, and that she would certainly use it while doing her job. She would also encourage others to use my strategy: spend more time on creating the solution and less time on arguing about the problem.

Speaking of solving problems, summer school that year was at a different high school. I needed to be driven across town to that school.

One day as Mom picked me up on her lunch break to take me home, she sighed, "This is quite a rushed schedule we have. I have to get you home and get right back to the office."

Before I thought, I said, "I take the bus." I almost wanted to take it back immediately, because the thought of riding the city bus all alone was scary.

Mom smiled broadly, "You could?"

I said, "Yeah, maybe."

She said, "Of course I'll show you how first. We will ride

49

together a few times over the weekend, and then you will be good to go on your own."

While I was learning to ride the bus, Mom had a sudden call to attend a meeting across the country. She left me in Dad's good hands to finish teaching me. He would drop me off at the school and then point to the bus stop and say, "You catch bus #61 right there and then get off in front of your old junior high school. You know how to walk home from that point."

I did not know it at the time, but he would come back and follow me to be sure I got off safely at my old school. He said that he became frantic when the bus stopped at my old school but I did not get off; I got off a few blocks farther down the road. Why? Because I realized that there was no crossing guard at the junior high stop during the summer, and there were signal lights at the other stop. I thought that would be safer for me to cross the busy street. Boy, was he happy to see me get off the bus, wait for the Walk sign, and then cross the street and head home as if I had been doing it all my life.

That was the first of many bus routes I have learned. I would say that I am probably the best bus rider in my family. One time when Mom was in charge of the trip, we got off the bus at the wrong place. Later, I will tell you about the two times I took a wrong turn.

The next summer, I was lucky enough to get an English class at my neighborhood high school. We talked to the teacher at the beginning of the session to let her know that we would be on vacation during the class and I would miss a couple of days. She agreed to give me the work I would miss, and I could do it while I was on the road.

But when I returned after our vacation, the teacher said I could not resume my place in the class.

"Why?" we asked.

"Because the computer has kicked you out of the class," she said.

"But people put information into the computer all the time; put him back in," we insisted.

But she explained that the computer had kicked me out, and out I had to stay. It was time to see the principal.

After some discussion with the principal, Mom asked me if I really wanted to be in that English class. I told her, "Not really." The principal offered me a place in a math class down the hallway, if that math teacher agreed and thought that it would work out for my level of math knowledge. Math is one of my strong suits, you know. I was getting excited about this move.

We walked down the hall and knocked on the math teacher's door. The principal explained that we wanted to join his class for the rest of the summer session without mentioning the problem with the English class. The math teacher asked me a few simple math questions, which I answered correctly, and I was in. I preferred math to English anyway. It was my stronger suit. It pays to have at least one strong suit.

It was nice that we did not have to waste valuable time discussing the problem with the English teacher. It no longer related to our solution at hand. I like peace and harmony. We did not need that information in order to work on a solution with this new teacher to earn some summer credit. Problem solved, credit earned; all's well that ends well.

Like my time in elementary and junior high school, the four years of high school just seemed to go by so very quickly. It was no time at all before I was donning a tux to have my senior picture taken and choosing a class ring; my ring was engraved with my full name inside, "Dean A. A. Poyadue," our school's name (good old James Lick High), our graduation year, 1995, and our class motto, "Reach for Tomorrow." What a perfect motto for me. I can't believe that they were able to engrave all that on one little ring, but they did. I looked at my brother's ring, and it does not contain all of that information. We were lucky to have a ring that held so much memorable information. Thank you, James Lick High and class of 1995, for choosing so wisely.

The next thing I knew, I was planning to escort the prettiest girl in the world (my sister Jill) to the senior dance. Weeks before prom night, I went through the school getting people to sign my yearbook. I was so excited, as people wrote all kinds of things in my book. Then one mean person came up, and after writing a few words, she took my book and ran away. I went home practically in tears. All I could say to my family was, "She took my book; she took my book!" We went back to the school to try and get some answers, but to no avail. The school leaders decided to just give me a new book. But of course, it was not the same, because all the nice comments from my classmates were gone.

So I do know that bad things can happen, and I know that there are bad people in the world. I also know that there are people that you cannot trust. I know I must use my good judgment skills to evaluate those I encounter in life. I am blessed with good judgment skills to help me decide whether someone is good or bad. Some people are very smart, but they have poor judgment skills. It's great if you can get both, good intelligence and good judgment skill, but if you can't get both, I think I got the better of the two possibilities. Making wise decisions can really pay off. I should probably say thank you to that girl who stole my yearbook; she sure taught me a good lesson, but boy was I mad and sad at that time.

Jill and I made quite a couple at the prom. I was the usual "handsome dude" that I am, and she looked like a beautiful princess. Even she was a little surprised at how popular I was; I even won two awards that night, one for dancing and one for most improved student. I don't know who was more anxious to get home and tell our parents what a wonderful evening we had, topped off by my two awards.

But the real highlight of my high school years came the evening of my graduation. When they called my name to walk across the stage to get my diploma, all of my classmates spontaneously stood up and applauded. Yes, Mom had tears in her eyes and my brother had the video camera pointing in the wrong direction. He never captured the moment. Like I said earlier, you can't always have it all your way.

So it was good-bye to dear old James Lick High—kind of sad, but mostly joy, happiness, and a lot of proud feelings.

My family threw me the usual graduation party. All my family and friends came. They all contributed to the two real live money trees that I had, if they preferred not to buy a gift.

Teacher Pat gave me one of the best gifts of all: a Dr. Seuss book entitled *Oh, the Places You'll Go!* I really liked the page that says, "You have brains in your head. You have feet in your shoes. You can steer yourself any direction you choose. You're on your own. And you know what you know. And YOU are the guy who'll decide where to go."

In the inside cover of the book she wrote, "Dean: I am so very proud of you. You have come a long ways, baby. Happy Graduation. Much Love, Teacher Pat '95."

I have tried not to disappoint her.

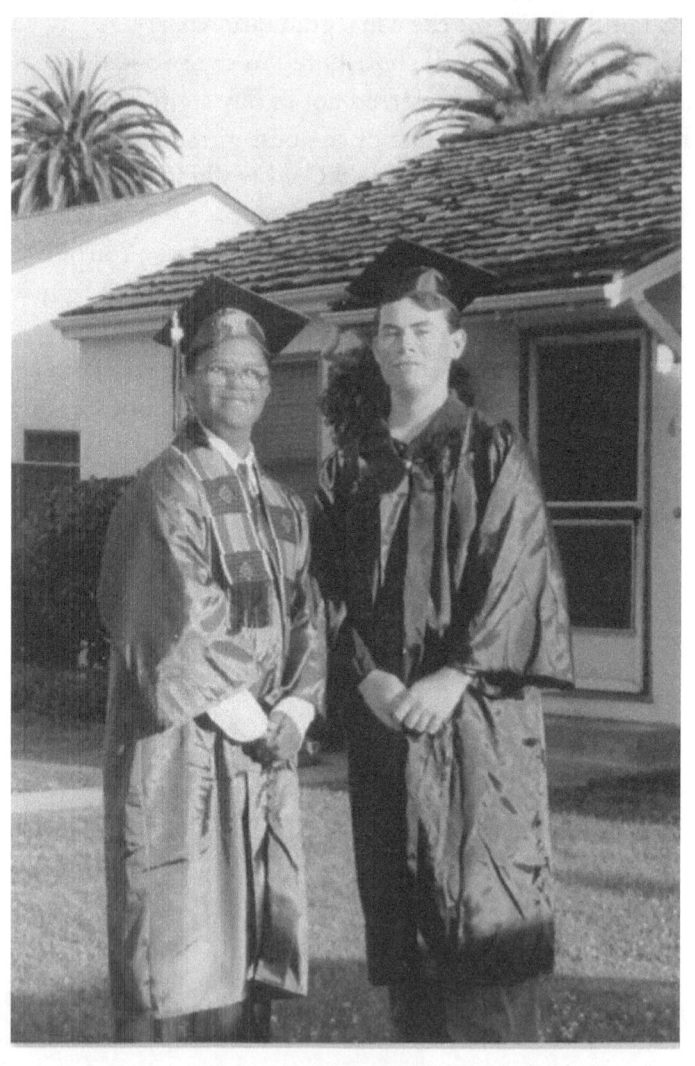

Chapter 5
19–21 Years of Age

A Four-Letter Word: Taft

After my high school graduation ceremony and my big party with all of my friends, family, and neighbors, it was time to relax a little bit. I counted the donations from my money-tree and wrote thank you notes to everyone, especially my four favorite old aunts: Margaret, Billie, Edna, and Evelyn. I knew they would be there cheering me on to greater things. They added up to almost four hundred years of living and giving fun, funds, and hugs. I went to the bank and added this money to the account my parents had started several years earlier – a gift to minors savings account.

After unloading my money-tree, I looked over the beautiful graduation cards people had given me at the party, and once again I saw the book from Teacher Pat: *Oh, the Places You'll Go!* I thought to myself, *"you got that right!"* That is another one of my favorite things to say. Oh, what a night that was in 1995! Of course Pete and I took a picture together in our caps and gowns. Pete had attended a different high school.

We took loads of pictures during my graduation ceremony and my party. Everyone munched on all kinds of delicious foods, and we enjoyed Mom's favorite orange sherbet and 7-up frappe.

My gift from Mom and Dad was a two-week train trip across the country, followed by a seven-day vacation cruise. We each had a small room on the train. There were facilities for taking a shower and getting dressed before heading to the dining car for breakfast each morning. After eating, we would usually head for the observation deck and look at all the wonders of America's vast and beautiful countryside.

My mom was surprised to see that in almost every state we passed through, there were signs advertising different casinos. With all those signs scattered around the country, she realized that she was not the only one who liked the ca-ching, ca-ching machines. As we traveled from San Jose to Los Angeles on the train, we enjoyed listening to live musical entertainment and choosing delicious food from a menu. It was just like being in a restaurant. We had fun reading, playing cards, looking out the window, just chatting with each other or friendly strangers, and participating in other family-friendly activities on the train.

We had to change trains in Los Angeles. Unfortunately, the train was delayed about six hours—we never found out why. Finally, early the next morning we were on our way to exciting New Orleans. We were heading for "Poyadue Country," where my dad and his family had lived many years. People living there did not think that our name was different or strange, nor hard to pronounce, as was often the case in other parts of the country.

There were several more long delays as our passenger train had to wait for freight trains to leave a crossing area before proceeding. We never realized that freight trains were more important than people; they had the top priority. Before we knew it, we were almost a day late for our hotel reservations in New Orleans. Thanks to our trusty cell phone, we were able to call ahead and let the hotel know about our problem; that call saved our rooms at the hotel.

Finally, and I really do mean fi—nal—ly, we arrived in New Orleans, my dad's hometown area. He had spent half of his youth in New Orleans and Bay St. Louis, Mississippi. We looked forward to relaxing in our hotel, but when Mom kicked off her shoes, she realized that the carpet was soaking wet. Mom and Dad called the front desk, and they were quickly moved to dry quarters; our wonderful stay in the great Crescent City began.

First thing the next morning, we headed for Café Dumond for some café au lait and beignets (a special doughnut treat). We then visited several old friends of Dad's and dined on okra gumbo and other great foods for lunch.

After my first lunch in New Orleans, we headed out to visit with Alan, Keith's best friend from preschool and elementary school. Alan was now married and studying to be a doctor at Tulane University. We spent a few hours with Dr. Al, his wife, and their young son in their small but welcoming apartment before we hopped back into our rental car to drive across the bridge to Bay St. Louis to see more family and friends.

Dad's cousin Betty worked at a casino in Bay St. Louis, and she pointed us in the direction of fun, entertainment, and their best restaurant for dinner that evening. Before heading out to dinner, we had a good time looking at the furniture and artwork Betty's husband Andrew created. He was a fireman, but he was sure artistic also. He gave us one of his favorite carvings, which was of the Holy Family at the manger. Mom likes it so much she displays it in the kitchen all year long, not just at Christmas time. I am sorry to say that Andrew has died, so we are now even more protective of his carving.

The next day, we went sightseeing in the good old bay. Now that I think of it, I have been to two Bay areas: Bay St. Louis, Mississippi, and the San Francisco Bay area. Both are great places to live, but they are very different.

We went to St. Rose de Lima Church, where Mom and Dad got married way back in 1956. It was a fairly small but unique church. It was the first time I had seen a painting of Jesus with a little color in his skin—he was painted a bit bronze. I liked it. I thought he looked a little like me.

It was raining really hard the day my parents got married. A lot of the older people said that rain on your wedding day means good luck and a happy marriage. I guess they got that right. My parents have been happily married for over fifty years. Their golden anniversary was a big celebration for sure, orchestrated by my sister, my brothers, their spouses and me. Mom had promised to let me walk her down the aisle and give her away when they repeated their vows, and that I proudly did. All the grandchildren had roles to play also.

In Bay St. Louis, I visited the grave sites of my grandparents and great-grandparents. We had to visit two different cemeteries because back in those days, they buried the Americans of African heritage in the "Colored Grave Yard," and white people were buried in another cemetery. My grandparents were all kinds and colors of people: black, white, Native Americans (Choctaw and Cherokee), French, and I don't know what all. Maybe that is why I get along so well with all kinds of people.

Some of the people in our family were Creoles. The delicious food we ate in New Orleans was Creole food. Dad's sister had recently put a new headstone on their father's grave. We took pictures of that and many other things. From looking at the headstones in the graveyard, it was strange to see the several different ways others had spelled our last name in the past; most of the time they had changed or rearranged the order of the last four letters.

Of course we had to go by 217 Citizen Street, where my dad grew up as a little boy. Grandma Gert had sold their home for about $7,000 around 1968. Wow! It is amazing how much less homes, food and many other things cost about forty years ago. Why, even our beautiful home in San Jose, CA only cost $26,000 then. Of course mom and dad were each making only $4.00 and hour. Grandma would be pleased to know that the new owners are really keeping up the old home place. Dad said that it looked better than he ever remembered it looking. We tried to go inside but the new owners were not home at the time. Unfortunately, the house was totally destroyed many years later by Hurricane Katrina, which did as much damage in Bay St. Louis as you probably heard about it doing in New Orleans.

I am glad that I got to see that old house, so now Dad and I can talk about his home when he was a boy: what it looked like, and how he used to sit on its long, covered porch chatting with his friends. When he was around seven years old, his mom thought he had pneumonia; she rubbed his chest with some kind of warm ointment, covered it with special healing leaves from their yard, and then laid him on a mat on that porch so that the sun could help cure him (people did not go to the doctor in those days, as easily and quickly as we do today). It must have worked, because seventy-five years later, he is still around, and he looks very good for an old man of eighty-two years. Besides that, his mom lived to be ninety-seven years old.

We ambled on across the street to visit Ms. Liza, a very close friend of my dad's family. She had lots of pictures to share and explained that she was keeping Dad's property, two vacant lots next to her home, cleared of excess debris. Besides, it was a great place for her, her children, and her grandchildren to have picnics and other family celebrations. Dad thanked her for her kindness. The people in the South did a bit more smiling and thanking each other. I also noticed that my dad called anyone just a few years older than he was, Mr., or Mrs., or Miss rather than calling them by their first names, as we often do in California. There goes that respect and southern hospitality thing again. My parents insist that we not call older adults by just their first name. They are still uncomfortable with that, even though they have been in California over forty years.

After a few days in Bay St. Louis, it was time to head back to New Orleans, where we visited my dad's old high school, Xavier Prep. It was so small compared to my high school, but Dad seemed really proud of it. He attended that school a couple of years and then returned to Bay St. Louis and graduated from St. Rose de Lima high school, another Catholic school. I think he had only twelve students in his entire graduating class. My mom teases him about how small his senior class was, because she had twice as many classmates in her graduating class from Lovejoy High in Lovejoy, Illinois. Just think, my class had hundreds in our graduating class.

We still had a few old friends of Grandma Gert's to visit (and I do mean old, they were eighty-five to ninety-five years of age), before we headed off to the next leg of our trip, which would take us to El Paso, Texas. And I certainly did not want to leave New Orleans without seeing their famous football stadium, the Superdome. After stopping at a few other tourist sites, we turned in our rental car and headed for the train station.

Our next stop was El Paso, where my parents lived for many years when the Army transferred Dad from Fort Niagara, New York, to Fort Bliss, Texas. They laughed when they recalled how they had spent their meager savings to go to Niagara Falls for their honeymoon, only to have Dad return to his army base and receive orders directing him to report to Fort Niagara. So, after their honeymoon, it was back to Niagara Falls to live. What a crazy world!

They lived in El Paso for almost ten years, and they made many friends among the people in the army and at Providence Memorial Hospital, where my mom worked as a Head Nurse. That meant I had a lot more people to meet and visit with on this exciting train journey.

I especially enjoyed the old museum at Fort Bliss, which displayed statues of their horses and showed the old uniforms soldiers used to wear. My parents took me to see some of the homes where they lived; the first year they lived in El Paso they moved six times, trying to find a decent house to rent. No one would rent to them because they were Americans of African heritage. Can you imagine, at that time it was legal for people to do that to other people? Sad.

We went to visit Mrs. Desboine, who was almost a hundred years old. She and her late husband were both high school teachers, African Americans, and had managed to buy a few pieces of property in El Paso. They rented Mom and Dad a very nice house, and Mr. and Mrs. Desboine and their three kids became a second family for my parents. They respected and loved the Desboine family very much.

Edna, one of the Desboine kids, had Down syndrome. Mom says she was able to take good care of me and help other parents because Mrs. Desboine had set such a good example of caring for and including Edna in everything. When I was born all those many years later, my mom's first thoughts were of Edna and her wonderful parents. See how things continue to circle around and connect? I told you about that before. And here those connections were again-- connections helping. "What goes around, comes around," so say the old folks. Mr. and Mrs. Desboine helped my parents, and now my parents were helping thousands of other families with children who have special needs.

There were other friends to visit, share a meal with, and share photos and stories. My mom had brought along a couple of bags of photos and albums to show them. Everyone we visited had photo albums and pictures displayed throughout their homes. It really was great fun meeting people from my parents' past. The people of El Paso were very friendly and eager to meet me. Many of them already knew something about me, and several even had pictures of me among the photos in their homes. It was amazing, some even showed us old copies of our family Christmas letters that we send out each year, and they said how much they looked forward to receiving them.

Mom also visited a couple of doctors she had worked with at Providence Memorial Hospital. We apologized for intruding into their very busy day, but they were happy to see Mom and meet us.

My parents were eager to try the restaurants in El Paso, since they were not allowed to enter them when living there between 1957 and 1965. You remember, the old African American thing. It must have been a strange world in which to live. I can't imagine my parents not being able to do everyday regular things, like going to a movie, a restaurant, or a bowling alley, or not being able to live anywhere they wanted. In spite of that, I noticed that Mom and Dad were visiting friends who were black, white, and Hispanic, and everyone greeted us with warm hugs. That was just like being in California now. It was a bit confusing.

In 1965 they left El Paso. My dad was stationed in Germany as one of his Army assignments and my mom and oldest brother, Turhan moved there to join my dad. My mom even worked in the army hospital. They felt free there to come and go, sit and eat as long as they had the money to pay. They talk about the dollar being very strong then. In order to help me understand, they said that one of our quarters could buy a dollar's worth of Germany's goods. Before we knew it, it was time to board the train and head back to San Jose, via Los Angeles (or so we thought). The train was late leaving El Paso, and that threw the whole connecting schedule off. The train engineer realized that we were going to miss our connection in LA and decided to drop us all off at a bus station, so we could meet the train in Santa Barbara, its first stop out of Los Angeles. Not a real swift idea.

We got to the bus station and, along with a bunch of other train passengers, grabbed our luggage and boarded a bus to Santa Barbara. Some of the passengers started to grumble about being hungry, so the bus driver stopped by one of America's favorite chicken places and bought a box of food and something to drink for each of us. My dad volunteered to pass out the food and drinks as the bus continued to bounce along as fast as possible, trying to reach the train's next stop before it arrived.

We missed the train again. Ugh! It had pulled into the station before we got there and did not wait for us. The bus driver continued on to San Luis Obispo, where we finally connected to the train and headed into San Jose, our hometown. That was about a three-hour ride. We never even got a letter of apology from the train folks. Other than the train problems, I very much enjoyed my trip halfway across the country. I met a lot of people and saw many, many interesting things.

And now it was time to prepare to go off to college. Whenever my family would say that I was going to Taft College, people would say, "Where is Taft College?" And for the fifteenth time they would say, "It is in Taft, California, about a four-hour drive from San Jose. The little town is named for William Howard Taft, the twenty-seventh president of the United States." We looked him up in the dictionary and learned that he was president from 1909 until 1913. He was also a Chief Justice of the Supreme Court, from 1921 to 1930. To be honest, we had never heard of Taft, California before, and we also did not know most facts about President Taft. We had increased our own education.

Believe it or not, there was one person who recognized the name Taft as soon as we told him that I would be going there to attend college. It was my pediatrician, Dr. Hyatt. He said, "Sure, I know Taft very well. I did my internship in Bakersfield, which isn't very far from Taft, maybe a thirty-minute ride. I also tried to rent an apartment in Taft, but to no avail. They cared not that I was a doctor, they only noticed my beautiful brown skin and would not rent to me. So as soon as I could, I moved to San Jose." He then gave me a hearty hug (you could seldom get away from Dr. Hyatt without a huge hug) and a manly handshake. He said, "Congratulations, Dean, I know you will do fine there, and I understand that things have changed a lot in Taft. It used to have a real negative image for people of color. If anybody can make it in Taft, it will be you, Dean."

I said, "Oh yeah!"

I was enrolled in Taft's very first Transition to Independent Living (TIL) class. One day, someone had called my mom at her office and asked her if she would evaluate a new program that Taft College was starting. The parent wondered whether to send her daughter to that program. My mom said sure, she would check it out, and she started to research the program. After a few days, she called the parent back and said, "I don't know whether you want to send your daughter there, but I am signing up my son for the first class, which starts in July."

That was her way of saying that she thought it sounded like

a darn good program. It was a two-year program at the junior college. Transition to Independent Living (TIL) students would stay in dorms that had been used by Taft's football players in the past (but they no longer had a team). The students would each have their own room in which they could have a small refrigerator, bed, desk, microwave oven, television, telephone, and bookcases. They would share a bathroom with one other student.

Their studying would start at 7:30 in the morning and end at 9:30 in the evening, five days a week. They could take whatever regular classes they could handle, including several core classes and special classes on learning how to live independently. The students would try several different jobs, including working in the library, the gardens, the kitchen, the cafeteria, and more. They would learn how to cook, do laundry, set up a bank account, write checks, create a budget, and pay their bills at the college. They would learn how to use transportation systems (buses, trains, and cabs) and how to set up doctor, dental, and other appointments. These were just some of the things they would learn.

Taft TIL students also learned the difference between "needs" and "wants." Many parents say they wish their children *without* special needs could have an opportunity to learn the difference between "needs" and "wants."

Of course, as prospective Taft students, we had to complete an application process and meet certain criteria before we were accepted into the program. Some of the questions included: had we completed a high school curriculum? Could we handle being on our own, away from our parents and the familiarity of our hometown? Could we follow instructions and be trusted to obey rules and regulations of the campus? No one was going to be watching us twenty-four hours a day. Of course, there was always a counselor on campus should we have a question or a problem.

After I was accepted, along with all the other students and their parents, we were invited to an orientation class. Mom said she knew it was going to be all right when she heard Jeff Ross, the coordinator of the program, say, "You are now Taft students;

we expect you to just blend in." Then he told us about the specific rules and regulations, and about our opportunities and responsibilities.

We spent the next few weeks buying stuff for my room. This was great: a new television, a keyboard (remember, I had taken piano lessons, even though I wasn't that great), sheets, a bedspread, a bookcase, a microwave oven, an iron, a tiny refrigerator, and of course some new clothes and shoes and a lot of other stuff. And yes, I took my video camera.

In no time at all, I had worked with the staff to get my phone installed, opened my bank account at a nearby bank, and created a budget for myself. I also became acquainted with the nearby regional center office; my records and case file were temporarily transferred there from San Jose.

Since I was now over eighteen years of age, I had started getting some Supplemental Security Income (SSI) funds. I applied for the SSI funds at the Social Security office. These are funds from the federal government to help poor or disabled people. SSI *is not* Social Security Administration funds. It gets confusing for some families because the Supplemental Security Income program is handled by the local Social Security Administration office, but it is not Social Security funding. I could use these funds to help pay for my education. To help us prepare to live independently, the school insisted that students go to the office, and not our parents, to pay our bills at the college. The regional center, a state of California agency that helps individuals with special needs, also provided some funds to help cover a part of my expenses. And like all college students, of course there was always good old Mom and Dad to provide for whatever else might be missing.

I was there just two weeks when I heard a knock on my door about ten o'clock one Saturday morning. Yes, it was Mom and Dad at the door. They said they were just checking to see if I needed anything. Before they could get settled in my room, there was another knock on my door. One of my friends was there with her tennis racket, asking if I wanted to play awhile. I looked at my parents, and they looked at me and said, "If you want to play, that is just fine; we can find a restaurant, have a little early lunch, and head back home to San Jose. It looks like things are going to be just fine here." And that's what they did.

I called them about five hours later to be sure they had gotten home all right (it's about a four-hour drive from Taft to San Jose). That was my first time calling to check on my parents; it felt a little strange. Just that same day, they had come down to check on me, and now I was checking on them. 'What goes around, comes around;'

I told you that before.

TIL students worked long, hard hours. We covered a lot of subjects related to independent living, as well as reading, writing, and math. We were also taught how to socialize, have fun, and relax as a part of a full life. I took full advantage of the idea of having fun when my birthday arrived on September 23. With permission from the Transition to Independent Living staff, I planned my twentieth birthday party. I had only been at Taft about three months, and I already liked and trusted the staff. They were all business-- but kind and caring. Together, we planned a great party.

I invited my whole class and also invited family from as far away as Los Angeles (actually Altadena, California) and Oakland. The party was held in the school cafeteria, which we decorated. Mom and Dad brought a cake from our favorite baker in San Jose, not knowing that the cafeteria staff was planning on making me a cake also. Needless to say, there was plenty of cake for everyone.

I always did like having a great birthday party. Sometimes, I would have two or three birthday parties with different groups of people for the same birthday. Even when I was little, I would have a party with my sports team, then one with my family, and one with my neighborhood friends. There might be a party for me in the nearby Catholic school's yard, where my sister and brother attended elementary school. Their classmates would buy me gifts, and we had cake during their lunchtime. That was real fun, but it was not my official birthday party. No one ever said you could only have just one party per birthday. Try it, I bet you will like it; don't do it every birthday, just some special ones.

If I were home sick, at the end of their school day, some of my brother's and sister's classmates would walk to our house and bring me get well cards. Our home was very close to the school. Besides meeting them at their sports games or the church fiesta, I had already gotten to know many of those kids by talking to them through our backyard fence while they were out for recess. Many years later, my little nieces and nephews had the same fun talking through the fence to St. John Vianney students out for lunch or recess.

After my birthday party at Taft, I gave all the family a tour of my room and enjoyed opening my gifts. What a great way to get launched into my first year at Taft College. My parents could hardly believe that so many people had driven such long distances for my twentieth birthday. Birthday number 21 is supposed to be the special one; we would surely have to put on our thinking caps for planning that one in order to top this.

My first year ended without a hitch. I thought everything went well. The first year report sent home to my parents was next to glowing. We were only given one month off for summer vacation. Taft meant it when they said this was a full two years of work and study. That was just fine with me.

When we returned from vacation, we realized that we were now the upper classmen, and there was a new group of beginners starting. After a few months of getting to know the new students, one of the girls "caught my eye," as the guys sometimes say. Her name was Kim; she was cute, smart, talkative, and very opinionated. She was from Santa Maria, California. She told me that her parents owned a vegetable farm called Babe Farms, where they grew small baby vegetables. I thought, *"Now here is a real babe from Babe Farms."* More later on Ms. Kim.

During year two at Taft College, we continued our intense classroom study and work performance program. We tried our hands at each of the several jobs that were being taught. I liked them all: working in the gardens, the cafeteria, the library, the shop, or whatever was offered.

We learned to cook, and we created a binder of healthy meal plans, which I took home with me and used during my bachelor days. We even had a chance to invite our parents down to eat one of the meals we had cooked. We learned to purchase tickets and catch the train or bus to go home and back to the college. I can't begin to tell you all they taught us; everything from being safe to making good decisions and avoiding bad ones.

The staff was very friendly and caring. They became well known to us, and we were well known by them. Don't hesitate to call Jeff if you would like more information about the program. Although he is the very head of the program, we all called him Jeff, not Mr. Ross; he had given us permission to do that. Calling people by their first names sure seems to be socially acceptable in California.

Kim and I both joined the basketball team. We were quite enthusiastic about the game. Our team played well enough to be in the finals. My dad videotaped our final game. He was so excited about the game that you can get a headache just trying to watch the video, because the picture is constantly bobbing around. I am sorry to report that we lost that game. We were number 2, but number 1 in our parents' eyes that year. We were still proud; we had tried.

Another kind of first did happen at that championship basketball game. Kim's family and my family met for the first time. My mom walked right up to Judy, Kim's mom, and said that I was interested in her daughter; she asked how she felt about that. Judy said she was open to Kim having a full life, including boyfriends and more. Since our families were from two different cultures; Kim was white, and was also born with Down syndrome. My mom wanted to be sure there were no negative issues to our courting on that account. She simply asked Judy if she had any problems with me being black. Was she okay with Kim thinking about getting married, if things should progress that way? The answers were - no problem, no problem with any of these things.

We may not have won that basketball game, but I thought it was a very successful day. Kim had a wonderful family, very much like mine. Judy and Frank, Kim's dad, loved their child very much, wanted a full life for her, and believed in her ability to be able to do. I think my good teachers at Taft helped parents believe in the ability of their children with special needs to do, and the program sure did live up to its name: Transition to Independent Living.

Three months into my second year, it was time to celebrate that all-important birthday #21. It was September 23, 1996. I had already told my parents that there were three things that I wanted to do on this birthday: go to Las Vegas and put three quarters in a slot machine (one at a time, of course), go see a girlie show, and have a beer with Dad. Sure enough, it was going to happen. Not only was it going to happen, but, old Aunt Margaret, my sister Jill, and her husband Roman were coming along for the fun and to sing "Happy Birthday" to me.

Aunt Margaret rode down to Taft with my parents in their old Buick to pick me up for the trip to Vegas. I introduced them to some of my classmates. Kim seemed quiet and shy when I introduced her to Aunt Margaret. She just talked for a few minutes and then went back to her room.

Then we headed for Vegas. Jill and Roman flew into Las Vegas and joined us at Circus Circus Hotel, which has a lot of things to entertain young people. For three days, we saw the sights, had a lot of fun, sang "Happy Birthday" several times, and ate lots of great food at the restaurants, and then we headed back to Taft.

All three of my missions were accomplished for that twenty-first birthday. As a matter of fact, I won about ten dollars with those three quarters in the slot.

Mom said, "You can continue to play."

I said, "No thank you, I just wanted to put three quarters in to see what would happen. I did, and that's it. You can have fun with the ten dollars and see if you can win something." I have not played again since then.

The girls on stage were beautiful, and I enjoyed that show

with my family. But the beer with Dad, after just one or two sips, I thought, *"You can have it; I will stick to my OJ or Coke."*

During my second year at Taft, several students (including me) were chosen to go to a conference in Bakersfield. We were chosen by the college staff according to our ability to handle checking into a hotel, finding our way to the conference rooms, and making it back to our rooms. I was really excited to be chosen to go on such a big adventure.

My parents kind of freaked out when they called the hotel and the front desk said that there was no Dean A. A. Poyadue registered. A quick call to my cell phone cleared it up; I was assigned a roommate for the conference, and the room was registered in his name. Many times I have said, "Thank God for cell phones." They make life so much easier and less scary for me, and my family. I keep my trusty cell phone with me at all times; and I make sure that I recharge it every night.

At the Bakersfield conference, we could attend three different workshops. I can't remember all of the workshops, but I remember Mom and I had a bit of a discussion about the third workshop that I chose. One option was a workshop on preparation for work; the other was on dancing. I chose dancing. Mom tried to steer me toward preparation for work. I insisted that I had two good "school-type" workshops, and this third one should be about that "fun" part of life.

In the end, she agreed; it was my conference, my learning experience, and ultimately, my choices. She agreed that I had made some good choices before. Besides that, she told me this with a smile in her voice; she was not angry, and I was very pleased.

I did not know it at the time I was at the conference, but after I graduated, I had the opportunity to sign up for classes at Goodwill, where I learned a lot about preparation for work, job interviewing, the importance of a good handshake, and more. That is another reason staying with the dance class was a good decision at that time.

Next, I had an opportunity to attend an independent living

conference with my whole class in Sacramento, the capital of California. It was about a two-hour ride from Taft. The conference offered all kinds of workshops and discussion groups, but the main thing I remember about that conference was waking up in a hospital with a big lump on my head.

While I was not looking at where I was going, I walked right through a very clean glass door. I shattered the door and knocked myself out, scaring everyone half to death. The school staff tried to call my parents, but they were busy having fun in Reno, and Mom did not have her cell phone on. By the time they finally reached my parents, I was awake, but with a big headache. After thoroughly checking me out, they decided I was okay but needed to be quiet the rest of the day.

I learned a lot that day, including "look where you are going," whether you are walking, running, riding a bike, or driving a car. Wherever you are headed, that is where your eyes should be focused.

As for my relationship with Kim, by now, we were an item on campus. Another classmate decided that he liked Kim also. He and I had a couple of heated arguments, which the staff learned about. The two of us guys ended up in Jeff's office to learn "better ways" of settling disputes, before our words would come to blows. We learned that actually it was Kim's decision. She would have to let us know what kind of relationship she wanted with each of us, and then we were to abide by that decision like gentlemen.

Darn it, Kim changed her mind more than a couple of times. We were on, and then we were off, then on and off again. That was frustrating. I decided to just "cool it." She did have the right to decide which one of us she was interested in, and I also had the right to decide if I wanted to hang around for her decision. While she had the right to her decision, she still did not have control of me, nor what I could or could not do in the meantime. I did not have to wait around for her decision. There were other cute girls on campus, and one really had her eye on me. In the end, Kim was by my side at my graduation from Taft.

What a great day that was, my graduation from Taft. My brother Keith came down to the college ahead of everyone else and gave me a haircut. That was unusual, because my mom always cut my hair. She also cut my brothers' hair and my dad's hair. She was the family barber, as her mom before her had been. I can't recall why he decided to come down and cut my hair, but it was nice having brother-to-brother time together. I think that it helped me be less nervous about the upcoming graduation ceremony. Keith and Dad also helped me pack my stuff that day, since I was leaving my dear old Taft.

All the students at Taft College, the regular students and the TIL special needs students, participated in the same graduation ceremony. It was a beautiful thing to see. When they called my name, I walked very proudly across that stage and a big yell went up from my family and friends. The camera lights were flashing. I felt like a hero or a superstar. There was a big party on the school grounds for all grads that same night.

As a gift for successfully completing our training (and no doubt as a continuing part of our learning to live independently), the school staff took us on a three-day cruise. I loved the cruise and was glad that Taft always helped us to know how to include pleasure and play in our lives. That cruise experience came in very handy, as my parents had planned a seven-day family fun cruise as my graduation gift. I was an experienced cruise traveler and had no trouble finding my way from my cabin to the clubs and back again.

The ship visited places like Venezuela and Aruba. I loved returning to the ship for dinner and the shows and dancing in the clubs. One of the bandleaders asked me to join her group and gave me a maraca to shake as she played guitar and sang. The next night when I entered that same club, she was on stage and yelled out, "Dean is here!" I sat at the front table and listened to the music for a while, and then she put her guitar down and asked me to join her in a dance. I think I told you before, ladies often asked me to dance, because I like to dance and I'm pretty good at it. But this was really something to smile about.

We had lots of fun that night, but then the ocean waters turned rough. They were tossing the ship around like a toy in a bathtub. I think my mom and I had less of a bad reaction to the churning of the sea than my dad because we were so busy dancing, while he was trying to lie quietly in the cabin and read. He was having a very hard time keeping his dinner in his stomach, and so was Aunt Peggy, my Uncle Stew's wife.

Uncle Stew was an old navy medic, and he had made all the arrangements for the cruise. He was having no trouble with the churning seas. He and Aunt Peggy have gone on many cruises. Sometimes, in the evening before dinner, we gathered for snacks and drinks in their suite, which had a balcony.

In the end, Dad actually had the last laugh on Mom and me, as she and I ended up with what they call "sea legs" when we returned home at the end of the cruise. We felt like the house was moving all around us. We had to head for our beds, and we suffered there too, as even the beds seemed to be moving. Dad was laughing and feeling fine.

It was hard to believe that my two years at Taft had come to an end, and here I was back at my parents' home in good old San Jose, known as the safest big city in the country. By the way, Taft turned out to be a great little town. I enjoyed my stay there: the restaurants, the movie house, the bowling alley, and the high school next to the college. But most especially, I liked the people of Taft. That included special clubs like Rotary that were very helpful. They were not only friendly but also did special jobs around the campus for students and the school; they were just great to know.

It was also hard to say good-bye to Kim. She still had one more year at Taft College. Now we would have to have a long-distance relationship. *Who knows,* I thought, *maybe she will change her mind again and decide that she likes that other fellow better than me.* Someone said, "Distance can make the heart grow fonder." Of course that heart would already have to be "fond" in order to grow "fonder." But I wondered if distance could also help one to forget the other person. I guessed that I would just have to wait and see; in the meantime, I would get started on living my more independent life.

Again, I thought about Teacher Pat and her high school graduation gift to me, the book, *Oh, the Places You'll Go!* Taft had been a new place for me to go and conquer; I did it! I did it! Now I would need to not only go home, but I would need to soon leave home for another new place. I had mixed emotions: sad to be leaving my friends and the faculty, happy to be graduating, and a bit anxious about what the next place will be like. Of course, I am Dean A. A. Poyadue: "Can do, at least I try."

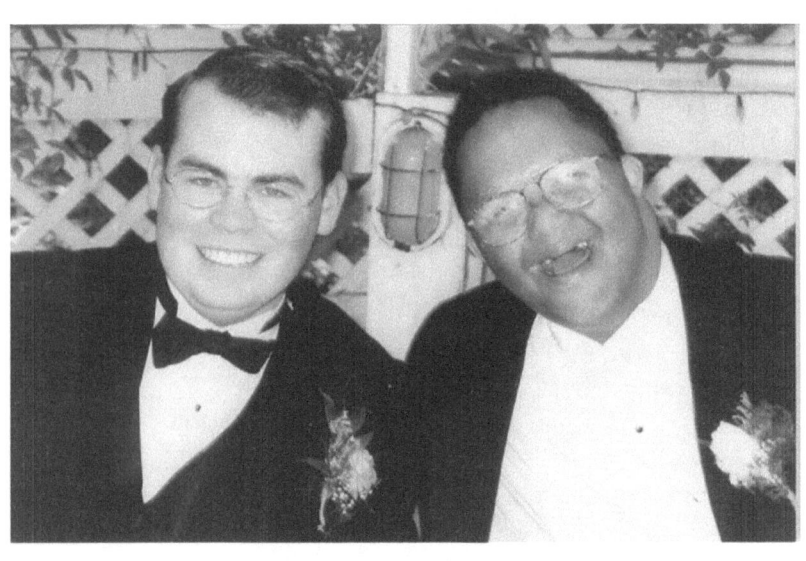

CHAPTER 6
BACHELOR YEARS

On My Own

Even though I had thoroughly enjoyed my stay at Taft, it was good to be home and back in my old bedroom. My room actually looked smaller than I remembered; it felt a little strange now that I was older and had been out of it for about two years. I loved catching up with my old friends, seeing familiar buildings and local landmarks in San Jose, and eating Mom's good cooking once again.

Being back home, I could walk right up to an old friend and say, "Wow! You haven't seen me for a while." Somehow, and I do not know why, but my greeting would get a special kind of chuckle out of them. They would smile and say, "Welcome back, Dean." The guys would give me a warm handshake, and most of the ladies would give me a very tight hug. I have noticed that some guys are beginning to copy the ladies, and they too are adding a bit of a hug to their handshake. That is nice. Anyway, by the smiles on all of their faces, when I said, "You haven't seen me for a while," I guessed that they really were thrilled to see me again, and I was certainly happy to see them.

If you have not had the pleasure and joy of walking through

the front door of your home and being smacked in the nose with a whole bunch of flavorful smells, you have not completely lived. I had missed Mom's famous spaghetti sauce, and on Saturday mornings, I loved the smell of great flaky biscuits, special applesauce-banana-walnut pancakes ("browned just right," was the secret to their delicious taste, she said); or the hint of cinnamon in her raison or French bread French toast. I had also missed our family's frequent outings for Chinese food, our favorite. The best thing about Chinese food is that there is almost always some left over to take home. And your good fortune may be that by the time you get home, your appetite and your stomach are both about ready for it.

I had some extra funds in my savings account that I had kept from birthday, Christmas, and other gifts (besides, I had had a couple of jobs while in high school). I decided that I would like to get some new furniture for my bedroom, something to match the new, more independent, manly me. So Mom, Dad, and I went shopping. It wasn't long before I saw just the bedroom set I wanted. It was a masculine, dark brown wood. I chose a queen-size bed for this king, a chest of drawers, and a dresser with a full-length mirror that could be placed at a couple of different positions. I liked to check myself out in the mirror after I was all dressed up, to be sure everything looked good. This mirror worked well for that. Sometimes when I'm checking myself out, I say to myself, as I pose this way and that way in front of the mirror, "Perhaps I should be a model." The bedroom set was to be delivered to my parents' home, but I knew it would not be long before I would be moving it into my own place.

I was 'liking summer time, and the living was easy,' cause I had no job yet. After a couple of weeks' rest from my hard work completing Taft's TIL program, it was time to start reconnecting with the helping agencies in San Jose and throughout Santa Clara County. I needed to talk to agencies that could help me move into my own place, find a job, and get to know whatever city I decided to live in (its public transportation, libraries, grocery stores, banks, restaurants, etc.).

Of course, the first agency we called was Parents Helping Parents – The Family Resource Center. Mom had learned early in my life that checking in with other parents who were a step ahead of you was always one of the best places to start. They would not only have up-to-date information on other agencies that could be of help, they would also be able to share with us the best way to approach them, and which ones to contact first, second, and third. We would waste much less time that way.

PHP's staff and its Adult Information Packet helped us connect with families who already had adult kids living away from home. Since most of their staff is also parents of children with special needs, they might have some answers for me. All of that would work well to give us a quick and more successful start.

Next, we called the regional center in order to set up a meeting to get a new case or care manager for me, and to put my folder back in the active files. I needed to put my folder back "on the front burner," as one manager used to say. The regional center's main job was to help pay for services and to make sure I was getting all the services I needed. They also wanted to be sure none of my rights were being denied, and I was being cared for just fine, in a safe and quality manner. Regional centers have a big job! They are private nonprofit agencies that carry out the State of California's commitment to ensure the care of individuals with developmental delays. I liked my old case manager, and I was sure that the new one would become a friend too. Some people like to keep their old managers forever, but I don't mind getting new ones. I like adding more and more people to my list of friends and helpers. The more friends I have, the happier I am.

We started to call other agencies that help individuals with special needs find and maintain their own independent housing. A nonprofit agency called Housing Choices was included on our list of calls; so was one called Greater Opportunities. It was important to gather as much information as we could from each contact we made. We never knew whether a particular person or agency would be the one to supply the specific answers we were looking for or to provide the services we sought; sometimes they could direct us not to 'the answer,' but to our next good source of information. By being in touch with more, rather than fewer, of them, we improved our chances for getting my needs met.

Besides that, they could also lead us to others who might help in our search for services, training, supplies, social activities, and many other significant pieces to complete my independent living puzzle, including finding a dentist for adults with special needs. Now that I was a man, I certainly did not want to continue to go to my children's dentist. By the way, my sister needed to find a dentist for adults with special "fear of dentists" issues. I did not need that, because I am just a little scared of dental procedures, not a lot. I can handle the dentist's office just fine, with my family there or by myself. I soon found a great dentist, actually two dentists— brothers named Peter and Paul. Their office was practically within walking distance of the new apartment and workplace I finally found.

During this searching process, we learned that when one person or agency says that they can't provide what you need, our next question needed to be, "Whom can you suggest that we might try next?" Smart people network like that all the time, whether they are trying to find a job, a painter for their house, a plumber, a doctor, or a car mechanic. Networking (or working the Net) was and is the name of the game for more success. Speaking of working the Net, I made sure Mom and Dad put a good printer, computer, and fax machine in my bachelor pad. I did not have to beg for those things because they knew that kind of technology would help make their lives as well as mine easier and less stressful. It was fun working with everyone to get me settled on my own. We all tried to keep an open mind and a positive attitude, and we hoped that all would turn out well in the end.

I finally got settled in lovely Sunnyvale, California. Sunnyvale was found in a recent study to be the happiest place in America. That was a perfect spot for an upbeat kind of guy like me. My favorite radio station was 949, so it was easy to remember my house address, because it too was 949. I was only about a half-hour car ride from my parents' home if I needed them to accompany me somewhere. Otherwise, I could just walk or take the bus and go about on my own. If I got lost, I would use my cell phone to call my family or friends to get me back on track. My family had talked to friends who lived nearby and asked if they were willing to be "emergency backup" if I needed something fast. I think we only had to use them once or twice. Thanks, Wayne!

We reconnected with the Department of Rehabilitation Services to get assistance with finding a job. We also connected with Goodwill Industries, which had a successful program for preparing people with disabilities for the workplace. The Department of Rehab attended a meeting with the Goodwill staff and me to decide on my work plan. The Department of Rehab paid Goodwill to provide me job preparation training. I immediately signed up for their next class on job preparation. Like I told you before, that really was an okay decision I made to take dance lessons instead of job preparation at that conference in Bakersfield while I was a student at Taft.

Since I was living in Sunnyvale, I had to catch two buses to get to the Goodwill facility in San Jose, where those classes were being held. I am lucky that I am a kinesthetic learner and not a visual learner. I learn best by doing things. I am a hands-on kind of guy. Mom is a visual learner, and she says that she and others like her have more trouble finding directions from one place to another than kinesthetic learners. Seems like there is always a little something for which to be grateful, even though I wasn't exactly excited about having to catch two buses a couple of times a week to get to and from class.

If my family did not have time to teach me a new route on the bus lines, there were people from the special needs service agencies who could do this. When it came to public transportation, Mom had given me one main rule to remember: "Only get off of a bus, or other public vehicle, at a place that you know or recognize, even if you have to ride around to where you first boarded. Do not get off in strange places!"

This rule came in handy one day when the driver did not hear the bell as I pulled on the cord to signal a stop to let me off. He went right past my stop. *What now?* I thought, *"don't panic, try to remember the one rule."* I kept looking out of the window until I saw something familiar. After many twists and turns of the bus, I saw Independence High School, where I had taken summer classes one year. I yanked hard on that cord and got off at the school. I knew how to get to my parents' house from there. It was a little far, but I walked home. "There goes another pound off my body," I smiled to myself. I sat on the front step and called my mom's office on my trusty cell phone. When Mom answered, I told her my story. She laughed and congratulated me on doing the right thing, and doing a very good job of handling and solving a problem.

She drove right over to pick me up and whisked me off to Goodwill for my class, after which I caught the bus again to get me back to my home in Sunnyvale. It was like getting right back on a horse after falling off. It is really hard to truly get lost when you and your parents are both armed with cell phones and pagers, as me and mine were. I blew an imaginary kiss to the cell phone and silently whispered a hearty thank you to modern technology for making living independently so much easier, less stressful, and safer. We noticed another strange thing: it was easy for me to learn to use most of the new technology stuff. As a matter of fact, my parents were more often asking me, than me asking them, how to do something on the cell phone, or programming the television, or some other piece of tech stuff. PHP has an Assistive Technology center called iTECH (introduction to Technology Easing Children's Handicaps); besides learning about computers at school and at home that was another place with low and high tech to help us special kids, our parents and/or professionals learn how to use technology.

Yes, all of this new technology available today comes in handy when one wants to live independently. For instance, if I received a letter that was hard to understand, I could just fax it to my parents, even as we were discussing it on the phone. We could make a decision about it right then and there. It was also fun to use my computer to send e-mails and print pictures of my nieces and nephews to post around my room.

I still have fun entertaining myself with video games or playing games with others; I also enjoyed playing my guitar. My keyboard somehow got lost in my mad rush to pack and leave Taft after graduation night. I haven't seen it since then, and my parents say they are not buying another one. I guess I will have to save for one when I start working. I can take time and save for it because I don't really need one, I just want one.

That was one of the really good things they taught us at Taft: sometimes you have to save funds in order to get something that you just want, but it is not a need, like buying your food or paying your electric bill. We learned that "wants" and "needs" are different, and "wants" can wait. I think that a lot of my regular friends should have taken that class where they went to college. They seem to buy a lot of what they just want, but don't really need, and then fuss about their bills that they can't pay.

I was sure glad that I still had my guitar when I returned from Taft, because I was really hooked on "country" at that time—country music, country clothes, and country entertainers; not so much these days. At that time, I wore cowboy boots, western shirts, and blue jeans. There was a specialty store where I shopped in downtown San Jose. The first time I went there, I asked the guy who was waiting on me for his card. That was just a habit of mine. I always ask for the cards of people who are working with me or helping me in any way. After that first time, I sought him out whenever I went back, and he always seemed to enjoy helping me shop. If anyone needs the phone number or address of someone who is assisting me with my independent living, I can usually give it to that person by just looking among my handy card collection.

Besides, it is just more businesslike. Yes indeed, I learned a lot at dear old Taft College.

I loved country music. Garth Brooks was my favorite singer, and my girlfriend Kim's favorite was Wynona Judd (she still is). Kim went to a couple of Wynona's concerts. She was lucky enough to get a chance to go back stage and get a hug, and now Kim's favorite computer screen cover is a picture of the two of them together. Nice lady, that Ms. Judd. Almost as nice as Neil Young and his wife Pegi who used to come to the San Jose area and help with a Christmas celebration fundraiser for children with special needs every year.

I often needed to get new heels on my boots because I did a lot of walking to places like the grocery store, and sometimes I walked to work, which was quite a distance. I also remember walking to restaurants, the dentist's office, shopping centers, the bank, the real estate office to pay my rent, the library, and other places near my home. Why, I can walk a mile or two very easily—without a huff or a puff. So I often needed to get new heels on my boots. And, wouldn't you know it, there was a shoe repair shop within walking distance of my apartment. I thought, *"My boots really are made for walking."*

It seemed like there was always something else to learn. That was good because that kept life interesting. By always learning, I had no time to be bored. Mom said that sometimes the people who worked in her office wanted to move on to another job when there was nothing more to learn about the job they were doing. "Always learning," sounds like a "good thing," as Martha Stewart would say. I wonder if Martha Stewart is related to my mom? Her name was Florene Stewart before she married my dad and became a Poyadue--just wondering; just thinking.

Community Association for Rehabilitation (CAR), formerly known as Community Association for the Retarded, provided job coaches for me. These individuals helped people with disabilities get acquainted with their workplace and helped the other employees and their managers know how to better work with employees

84

with special needs. CAR staff known as job developers also went out into the community to work with businesses to create job opportunities for individuals with special needs. CAR was happy to get involved in my independent living project, and right away they assigned a job developer and a coach to help me get started on my first real job.

By the way, I am glad that CAR changed its name from "Association for the Retarded" to "Association for Rehabilitation." When I was younger, Mom wrote to an office in the state capital to tell them that they could save themselves money, and save her and other families some heartache, by changing the name on their facilities. Mom suggested they simply put "Developmental Center" on their building. There was no need for the words "for the Retarded." They are now just called developmental centers. Little things can mean a lot and can save money too.

This must sound like a lot of calling and coordinating to get me started on my independent living. It was. It took time and energy. There was quite a bit to do to launch me into my own independence. My mom still called it interdependence, which she felt was the way most, if not everyone, in the world lived, especially if they had a full and happy life with family and friends involved, or to call on now and then for help or to share happy events.

It also took my parents' time, money, and energy to help launch my sister and brothers into their own homes. Many adult children need help with the down payment on their first home. And it certainly takes time and energy to help them by caring for grandkids. Besides being fun, being family definitely takes time and energy, I guess.

Speaking of family, at this point, I am not sure I want kids. "That is a *big* responsibility," I just came right out and told Mom one day when we were in church. I had been noticing some little kids making noise and not paying attention, even when their parents tried to get them to sit still and be quiet. Also, my parents would let me take care of my little nieces or nephews while they put dinner on the table. It was hard keeping up with them and keeping them from hurting themselves.

Later, when I brought up the subject of having kids, my parents said, "If you don't want the responsibility, then don't have children." They told me that there is nothing wrong with deciding that you do not want to have kids. It would be wrong to have them if you did not want them and could not care properly for them. I was relieved to learn that I did not have to automatically have kids. I could have a girlfriend, or a wife, and no kids. That sounded great. That sounded like something that I could definitely handle. Later, after Kim and I became engaged, the genetic counselors and doctors at Kaiser Permanente helped me to understand more about this "having kids" thing. They were great. Kim and I took classes about birth control. She decided to take the pill, but it started to affect her health. I decided that I could handle having a vasectomy.

I was learning all kinds of new things as we set up my independent living. Taft College had assigned a follow-up coordinator to help guide its TIL graduates for the first five years after we left school. My follow-up person was named Jaima. I don't know how she did it; she had a very busy schedule. She was always on the road, driving from city to city, across this big state of California to attend meetings, check on us, and visit with our parents to help us get launched and successfully settled. She helped us get appropriate homes, jobs, and other services to make our transition to independent living just a bit easier. She worked with all of the same agencies that my parents and I worked with. We all worked together. In that way, Taft could help us and, at the same time, gather information to evaluate how well their program was working and decide what needed to be changed, enhanced, deleted, or added to the TIL program. Jaima said since our class was the very first class, it was even more important for them to see how successful we were. Wow! That is another big responsibility for me.

Greater Opportunities was another agency we contacted. They were very helpful. They created various types of housing possibilities for individuals with all types of special needs. Some of the housing opportunities they offered were apartments, and some were single-family homes. Most of them were in the communities where their clients' families already lived. One of my classmates from Taft, Jason, and I decided that we would like to find a place to share. Jason and I were not 'great' friends at Taft, but we got along just fine, and our parents already knew each other, and he lived nearby in this Santa Clara County area also. That made it easy for his parents and my parents to work together to get things moving in the right direction for us. It took half the effort to find a place with four parents looking instead of just two; and our friendship grew during the process.

One day soon after we started looking for a place to live, Greater Opportunities called to say that they had acquired a five-bedroom home; they asked if we would like to take a look at it. Jason and I could rent it with three other guys. We would each have our own bedroom. This was great news, because some of our friends had to share a room. It was a lovely home on a quiet tree-lined street in Sunnyvale; it had a big living room, a cozy kitchen, two bathrooms, a great backyard with fruit trees, and a large patio for having parties and fun. Jason and I were the first to see it. We loved it! We decided right away that we would like to move into the two bedrooms downstairs as soon as we could get our stuff out of our parents' homes.

In less than two months after graduating from Taft College, I was out of my parents' home and had moved into my own place. The new bedroom furniture that I had recently purchased fit just fine in my new room. It was fun meeting the other three guys who were moving in with us. We all became good buddies. We respected each other's privacy, but we also did many fun things together like going bowling, going to Great America amusement park, or going to hockey or baseball games. Different families and different family members took turns getting us to and from these major events. We each prepared our own meals. We sometimes decided to eat together and would often order in pizza or go get Chinese food at a nearby restaurant.

We also had fun at each other's family affairs. For instance, we all gathered at my parents' home before heading out to have fun at our St. John Vianney Church fiesta. Our parents were great at dividing up assistance as needed and sharing expenses or driving duties. It just seemed to flow and work out without a lot of planning and discussion. No one was keeping an exact tab on who did what for whom, and how much each item cost.

We also threw parties at our own house, our bachelor pad, and we went to parties at other group homes or at special holiday events put on by Goodwill. Sometimes I went to mass with Mom and Dad on Sundays. Afterward, we would head out to breakfast at a nearby restaurant. This was Mom's one day off from cooking breakfast. While we waited for our food, we often discussed any problems or concerns we had. I often brought my bank statements and other mail with me, if I had any questions about them.

I even threw my sister a birthday party at our bachelor place. It just happened to be the same day that a local television station called my mom to see if they could interview her about her work with special kids. She said, "Sure, if you don't mind doing it in the middle of a birthday party." They came early to the party, interviewed several of us, and stayed until the party was almost over, having fun and learning more about the good life we were living. They were very interested when I showed them the schedule we had created for our daily routine and explained how we shared the home without major problems.

The television crew finally had to leave so that they could prepare the presentation for the evening ten o'clock news. It was fun having the party and then, a few hours later, watching it on the news. It was times like that, that I would remind my family that I still wanted to be a model or try acting. Maybe one day I would have that kind of job.

For now, my first job was as a stocker at a Payless store. I had to catch two buses to get there. Jason worked just down the street at a drugstore. Soon my job developer found me an even better job, with more hours, as a sales associate at a Michaels Arts and Crafts store. My good luck, I only had to catch one bus to get to Michaels. And on bright sunny days, I would start walking to the bus stop and just keep right on walking until I was at work, and some evenings, I would walk back to my home. I always left home plenty early in order to have time to walk to work.

I really enjoyed working at Michaels. All the people there were very friendly and helpful, and they encouraged me to be the best sales associate I could be. I kept busy doing many different jobs, such as stocking the shelves, unloading supplies from delivery trucks, helping customers find items in the store, keeping the store neat and orderly, and helping my coworkers. I was needed all over the place, and everyone liked my help.

Most of the time, I worked from nine o'clock until three o'clock, with a half hour off for lunch. There were plenty of places to eat nearby, so I seldom took a lunch to work (unless my money was getting low). When Michaels had a party at some fancy place, one of the employees would pick me up at my house and return me there at the end of the evening. They would always check with my parents to be sure that it was okay with them. I would use my trusty cell phone to call my parents to let them know when the other employee had picked me up, and again when I was home safe and sound at the end of the evening. It all worked out just fine.

I could not wait for my girlfriend, Kim, to come up from Santa Maria to see my new place. We talked on the phone and she said that her mom was willing to drive her up soon, on a Saturday. Her mom travels quite a bit for her business. So we had to wait a few weeks. It is about a four-hour drive from Santa Maria to Sunnyvale, but they finally made it up one Saturday. I invited my sister Jill and her husband Roman to join Kim, her mom, my parents, and me for lunch at one of my favorite restaurants. After lunch, Kim and I went to a nearby movie theatre, while my parents took Kim's mom to see the Parents Helping Parents Family Resource Center. Although its main services are to Santa Clara County, it also serves the rest of the state and nation as well. It is located about twenty minutes south of Sunnyvale.

After the movie, I took Kim across the street to an ice cream parlor for a treat, and that is where our parents picked us up to head home. The day went by much too fast; all too soon, it was time for Kim and Judy to head back to Santa Maria.

Kim was on her summer break from classes at Taft College. Soon she was back in school, and it was back to e-mails and phone calls for us. It wasn't long before it was my parents' turn to drive me down to Taft to visit Kim; we had lunch and then headed back to our part of California, back home toward San Jose. "Do you know the way to San Jose?" We did, many times. I guessed that this was what they called a "long-distance relationship."

I had graduated from Taft in 1997. My family and I drove down to Taft to attend Kim's graduation in 1998. That was another fun night of hugs, good food, dancing, and celebration. My family and I spent the night there in a hotel, and then we drove home the next day. I can't believe it, but this driving back and forth between Santa Maria and San Jose continued for five years.

As we approached the year 2000, people were making a lot of fuss about the end of the 1900s. My immediate and extended family in California was excited about being in charge of planning the Stewart-Walker Family Reunion for this year 2000. It was to be a big affair with family members coming from all over the country. The main event was to be held at the downtown Hilton Hotel. I told Mom that I wanted to invite Kim and her family to the reunion, where I planned to ask Kim to marry me. Mom said that she thought it was a fine idea, saying that she would have a champagne toast to our engagement done at the main event.

When I asked Kim if she was still interested in getting married, she said yes. That was not my proposal; I was just checking to see if I should even be thinking about proposing. You might remember that Kim often changed her mind. All was right with the world; she had said that she was still interested. I would make the formal proposal of marriage during the three-day family reunion.

So Mom and I went shopping for the perfect ring. We found it at the Post Exchange store at Moffett Field, a naval air base in Mountain View (between San Jose and Sunnyvale). They have an historic airplane hangar there, which Dad took me to see when I was younger. He worked at NASA there. We also went to the exciting Blue Angels airplane shows there as well. My dad, a retired soldier, still liked to "shop on post", as he stated it. Actually, I liked shopping on post also. Since I have an Army I.D. card, as an adult child of a retired military person, I can shop on post and also get health care. As a bachelor, I often shopped for my groceries in the commissary store located there. I am quite proud of my Army I.D. card.

Although I called Kim on the phone, asked her to marry me, and she said yes, and even though we had the champagne toast announcement of our engagement at the family reunion, I still insisted on getting down on one knee to ask her to marry me and properly present the ring to my girl. So, on the third day of the reunion, when we were having the family picnic in the park, I gathered all the family around. I asked Kim sit on a bench; I got down on one knee, and officially popped the question. She said yes, I put the ring on her finger, and now all was right with the world again. I had carried out my proposal the way I had always planned it. Yeah!

The night before the family reunion picnic, when we were celebrating our engagement with our champagne toast, Kim and I performed in the Family Talent Show: we did a country line dance. Everyone loved it, and we were asked to do an encore, which we gladly performed. We both love dancing, and if I must say, we did a great job that night. It seemed like everyone was in a mood for dancing after our toast: the three-year-olds and those ninety-three years young.

Speaking of the Family Talent Show, I must tell you a secret about my mom. She cannot tell a joke. And would you believe it, she chose to tell a joke for the talent show. The trouble was that she started laughing so much just thinking about the punch line, that she could not get the words out of her mouth. In the end, she got the crowd to laugh anyway; they were all laughing at her, because she couldn't stop laughing.

Our family, like a lot of families, has plenty of talent. Uncle Stew showed off his autobiography, which he had just written. He said he was giving the first autographed copy to me because I was always the first to return my registration form and my check whenever he sent out the reunion announcements. I felt so proud and thanked him for the book. Uncle Stew also made beautiful music with his clarinet; my sister-in-law Sara sang several beautiful songs; my nephews William and Jay Quinn both sang and played the drums; and Jay also did a little juggling act.

It was great to see Aunt Liz and Uncle Ben from Venice, Illinois, at the reunion. Whenever I go visit my mom's hometown of Lovejoy, Illinois, I always stay at their home, where there is plenty of good food and special treats. I was so sorry that Aunt Shoo-Shoo Lou-Lou was unable to attend. She is one of my favorites, because she also likes to dance, and she never forgets to call me on my birthday. Of course, I try to remember to call and sing "Happy Birthday" to her on her special day. Her son-in-law and I got along great, because he was the disc jockey at the last reunion and invited me to assist him; how exciting and cool!

It was a great three days of fun for all of us. I sure hated to see it end, and I asked Uncle Stew when the next reunion would be held. He said it would be in about two years back in his part of the country in Maryland, not too far from the White House and many other historical and interesting things that I could visit and see. You are right: Kim and I were the first to reply, and we attended that next reunion as husband and wife. But wait, I'm getting ahead of myself again.

After our engagement, Kim's parents, Judy and Frank, asked me to spend the week with them at their family cottage at the lake. Most of her immediate family was there for their summer vacation. That included her brother Jeff, his wife Kellie, their son Eddie, Kim's Aunt Terrie, and her friend Patti. Her other brother,

Brad, was in New York, performing. He was dancing in a show on Broadway and could not make it. He is a fun guy to have around, when he can show up, and he will often perform an exciting dance routine.

I must admit that I was a bit nervous about meeting Kim's dad again, although he had made me feel quite at ease when we had dinner together with her grandparents in Santa Maria. As soon as Frank had entered the restaurant, he walked right over to my seat and extended his big hand and took my shaky hand; shaking hands man to man. And he quietly said, "How are things, Dean?" I think that I got three of my favorite words out: "Oh, just fine." It seemed that he respected me as the man who was about to marry his precious Kim.

I came to like Frank and to respect him as a man of his word, but a man of few words. He was going to be my father-in-law, and I liked the idea of having two fathers and two mothers. If one of each was great, wow, two would be twice as good. I always proudly announced to my family members who were meeting him for the first time-- "Frank is my father-in-law." It seemed like there were always more women around than men, so that was another reason I was glad to add another man to my life.

It took a whole year to plan our fabulous wedding. Our two moms were in constant touch, phoning and driving between San Jose and Santa Maria. Kim and I were pretty busy also. We spent a lot of time talking to the priest at the Santa Maria Catholic Church. We spent a weekend at a conference retreat house taking a class for couples preparing for marriage. There were about 20 other couples there; all of them were kind and helped us enjoy and 'get through' the process. After successfully completing everything that rainy weekend, the conference leaders gave us a certificate to take back to the priest at our church. Then there were engagement photos to be taken. Kim's mom took a playful set of pictures at the beach, and my mom had a more formal set of photos taken at a portrait studio. Our two moms sure worked well together.

It seemed like there was always one more thing to plan or to do to prepare for our big day. One of the hardest jobs was limiting the number of people we were inviting to the wedding. Family friends were calling our moms, asking if they could be squeezed onto the list. The church was big enough to hold many, many people, but they would also need to have a place at the reception, which had limited space. And we would need to feed them at the reception. We did our best to include as many family and friends as possible.

Kim and I also had to decide who would be in our wedding party. I always knew who my best man was going to be-- Pete, of course. And I was just as sure that I would be his best man when he finally found his special girl. About five years later, I was his best man when he married his sweet Abigail. Along with Pete, I chose Jason, a friend from my church, and my longtime friend Duane, and then I added my oldest brother Turhan as my final groomsman.

My brother Keith and his wife, Dana, were expecting their first baby around the same date as our wedding day, so we did not include him in the wedding party. As luck would have it, their beautiful daughter, Tayelor Marie, was born at the same moment that Kim and I were saying our "I do's" on August 11, 2001. We can never forget her birthday, even if we tried. And when she is older, she will always remember Uncle Dean and Aunt Kim's wedding anniversary. I think my parents were going crazy with happiness that day.

For her bridesmaids, Kim chose my sister Jill, her sister-in-law Kellie, and another Kellie, her best friend from Taft College; her childhood friend Diana was her maid of honor. Kim's two brothers, Jeff and Brad, were our ushers. We chose my four-year-old niece, the cute little Antonia Symone, to be our flower girl, and Zachary, my friend Pete's handsome nephew, to be our ring bearer. My nephew, Jay Quinn, and Kim's brother Brad were our readers.

Kim and her mom had lots of work to do: choosing color schemes, finding places for special events, picking out dresses for the wedding party, hiring entertainers, and sending out invitations—all the things that brides, and parents of brides and grooms have to do to create a wonderful wedding and a memorable reception. They even had a wedding coordinator to help them. With all of this attention, Kim and I felt very special and very loved, not special needs, just special people –really loved. Hopefully, all of this would lead the bride and groom into a full, long, loving, and happy life together. I kept thinking, *our life together is going to be as exciting and fun as this wedding.* I will jump ahead with a little secret for you: so far, we have been together ten happy years.

Our wedding rehearsal went well, and so did our rehearsal dinner, which was attended by about one hundred people. It was great! Because many of my family and friends had to travel long distances by car or plane, they had to get hotel rooms, so we decided to invite them to the rehearsal dinner. It seemed like everybody was excited and wanted to be involved in everything, which made it that much more fun for Kim and me.

Since we were getting married on August 11, our rehearsal dinner fell on my sister Jill's birthday, August 10. We thought it only right to include a birthday cake for her, and everyone sang "Happy Birthday" to her. We actually had two celebrations for the price of one. We were "Feeding two birds with one piece of bread," as mom insists (as opposed to that old saying "killing two birds with one stone").

Guests at the rehearsal dinner took many pictures, and several people made heartfelt or funny speeches, like the ones I make at our family reunions. Although I am a guy of few words, I always make a little speech at family gatherings. Then it was time to break up the party so everyone could get a good night's sleep before our very big day. Of course Pete and I had a hard time falling asleep, but the next morning we were up early and nervously preparing ourselves for my big day. Pete was a perfect best man, helping me with everything.

On the day of our wedding, the church was beautifully decorated, the sun was shining, and the weather was terrific – not too hot, not too cold. As everyone was being seated, to get the show on the road, my favorite singing sister-in-law, Sara, played the piano and sang a song I had requested: "From This Moment." It was the same song she had sung at Keith's wedding two years before.

As Sara sang, our guests filled the church. Kim's two brothers escorted our parents to their seats. Our two moms did a little candle lighting ceremony, indicating that our two families were being joined. The bridesmaids and groomsmen entered, as well as the flower girl and the ring bearer. Then it was time for everyone to stand and watch the beautiful bride come down the aisle on her dad's arm. Frank handed Kim off to me, and we both nervously climbed the few steps toward the priest on the altar.

Our regular priest was out of town on our wedding day, but we really liked the priest who conducted our rehearsal and performed our wedding ceremony. He was patient, kind, and funny at times. He kept us relaxed and enjoying what was happening. At one point in the wedding ceremony, he made everyone in the church laugh when he let all of them in on a little secret: Kim was giving him a hand sign to speed up the ceremony and get it over with.

We both thought that he would never get to that "You may now kiss the bride" part. First we had to hear his words, and listen to the readings, and hear some more lovely songs being sung just for us.

We left the altar and placed a beautiful bouquet of flowers near the Blessed Mother side of the altar, and then we exchanged hugs with each other's parents and headed back to the priest on the altar. F-i-n-a-l-l-y we heard, "I now pronounce you man and wife," and the "You may now kiss the bride" moment had finally come. As we turned to face the congregation and leave the altar, we showed our broadest smiles (of relief) as the priest continued, "I now present to you Mr. and Mrs. Dean A. A. Poyadue." The other singer strummed her guitar and burst into song, singing "I Believe I Can Fly" as we slowly made our way down the aisle and rushed out of the door into the warm, wonderful, welcoming sunshine.

Whew! It was over. The mass and the ceremony were really over, and we greeted family and friends before eagerly making our way into our waiting stretch white limousine. It looked a block long; it was beautiful and just what I had hoped for. After the traditional ride around town and a sip of champagne, we rode to our reception, where a huge wedding cake and hundreds of family and friends awaited us.

But before any fun or food, the photographer was also awaiting us, demanding that we turn this way, and that way, and take photos with this group and that group. I was getting hungry and so was Kim. When we thought that we could not stand to take one more photo, the wedding coordinator finally called us to line up for our big entrance into the reception. The DJ announced the wedding party's names, and then it was time for that "Mr. and Mrs. Dean A. A. Poyadue" shout-out again.

It felt good to take our seats at the center of the head table and have our food finally placed in front of us. Both Kim and I can enjoy a good meal any day. I think people believe that brides and grooms don't get hungry, well we sure did. As we looked out at the crowd of people there, they seemed as happy as we were. Pete's father Jim, our very good family friend and a priest, came to the front area to say a blessing for our food, after which he gave everyone the good news that Mom and Dad's third grandchild, Tayelor Marie, had been born. Baby and mother were both doing just fine. What a great day!

A special singer sang us a love song, and then Pete, my best man, gave a fitting toast about our long friendship and how he knew Kim must be the right one for me because I was always talking about her. He also said that he was sure that ours was a union that would last a long time. Pete did a great job as usual: he made it short, sweet, and snappy. Kim's mom and my mom had created a short video of each of our lives, and after that was shown, it was time to cut the cake and feed it to each other.

We fed each other cake; followed by the champagne toast. For the toast, Kim and I interlocked our arms at the elbow and then started to sip from the glasses, but she could not reach her mouth. So she got a real laugh from the guests when she used her other hand to take the glass from our entwined arms and successfully had a sip; the toast was completed.

And now, to the center stage: the dance floor awaited Kim and me for our first dance as Mr. and Mrs. Then Kim danced with her dad, and I danced with my mom, followed by the wedding party, and then all the guests joined the floor and danced for hours. Kim's brother Brad, the professional dancer, and one of his favorite dance partners, did a special performance for us. We still get very excited just looking at the videotape of that day, especially the dancing.

Yes, I did remove and throw Kim's garter to the eligible bachelors. My friend Duane was the lucky catcher. Kim then tossed her bouquet to the eligible ladies, and my childhood friend Gaby, who had travelled all the way from Palo Alto, was so excited as she clutched the flowers and looked around the room several times, as if to say to everyone, "See, I got it, I must be next!" (Kim and Gaby graduated from Taft College the same year.) Then my childhood friend Andrea (I liked to call her my "old girlfriend") led most of the guests around the reception area doing a conga line dance. (In just a few years, Kim and I danced at Andrea's wedding reception in lovely Santa Barbara, just a few miles down the road from Santa Maria. I totally interrupted Andrea's wedding ceremony by fainting right in the middle of it. The church was quite hot, but everyone teased me, saying that I was trying to stop my old girlfriend from getting married. The priest would not continue with the ceremony until my mom told him that I was just fine.)

I don't know if it was because the music was so great, or the people were in such a festive mood, but our guests continued to dance until about ten o'clock that evening. The reception finally started to grind to a halt, even though we had started it quite early in the day. My mom had already said good night an hour earlier, because our beautiful flower girl, Antonia, had "wilted" and needed to get some sleep. Kim and I were finally driven to the historic Santa Maria Inn for some much-needed rest.

The next day, we had a gift opening party in Kim's parents' backyard. There were all kinds of wedding gifts, large and small, including many checks, large and small, to create a nice nest egg on which to begin our lives together.

After the gift opening gathering, we headed home to pack, because the next day, we would be off to board a cruise ship for our honeymoon. Kim's brother Brad and his dance partner friend were also taking the cruise. It was nice knowing that they were on board the ship just in case we needed anything. Of course, I had been on cruises twice before, so I was used to being on a ship. As I have said before, I am pretty good when it comes to finding my way around a town or a ship. You remember that point about us kinesthetic learners often being good with directions and finding our way to and from places, and visual learners, like my mom, often getting lost.

The four of us enjoyed our time together, taking part in the ship's many fun activities. And Kim and I enjoyed our personal time alone, the many dance floors at the ship's clubs, and the nightly entertainment. Neither one of us tend to get dizzy or seasick. Before we knew it, the honeymoon was over, all too soon. The old folks were right once again: "Time flies when you are having fun."

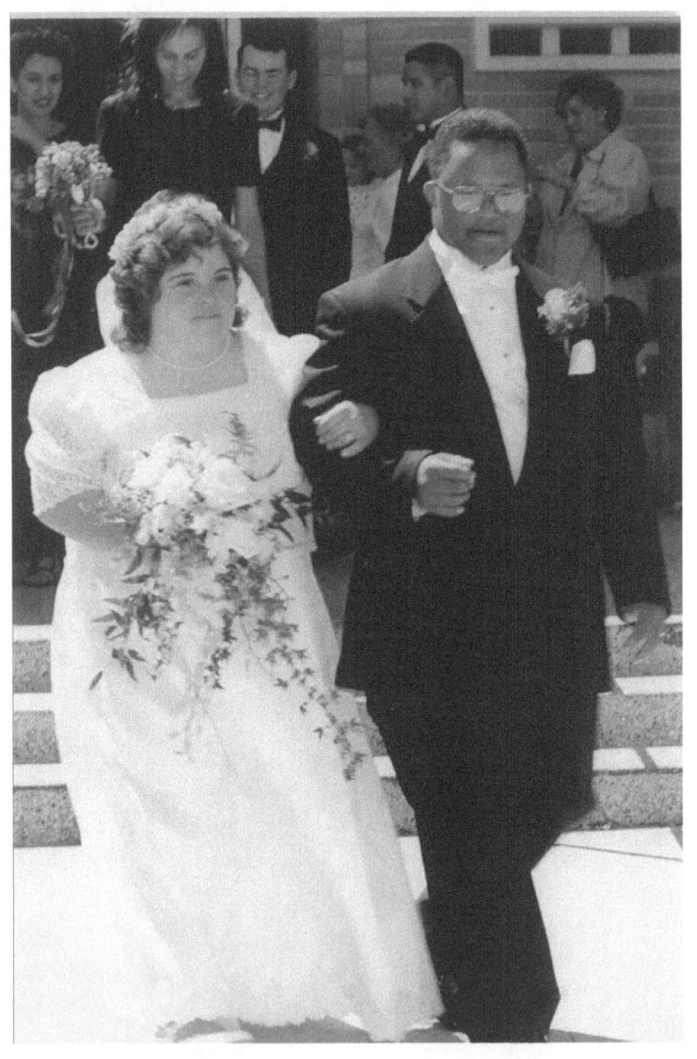

CHAPTER 7
FOREVER AFTER YEARS

Independent—But Not Alone

As soon as we were back from the honeymoon cruise, Kim and I had to separate. I needed to return to the apartment in Santa Clara that I shared with Jason. About a year before, we had moved from Sunnyvale after I won a lottery to get a brand new apartment there. The apartment was closer to my parents' home in San Jose, but much farther from my job at Michaels Arts and Crafts store in Sunnyvale, which I intended to keep, and I did.

Anyway, I now needed to go home and make arrangements to move my furniture and other things to Santa Maria. Kim and I had discussed where we would live. She decided that she did not want to move away from her family. And I felt that "a man's gotta do what a man's gotta do." That meant I was moving to her part of California.

Our parents had added their thoughts to where we should live. They thought that perhaps we should live near my parents first, because my parents are older and might not be around as long as Kim's parents. Later, we could move to Santa Maria near Kim's family. But they listened to us and accepted our decision. After spending a few weeks looking for a suitable apartment, in the best location, we decided to just move into the very nice two-bedroom apartment that Kim was already occupying. It was the same one that she had shared for a brief time with a girl friend after graduating from Taft College.

It was a good thing they did listen to us, because God is in charge of when we live and die. It just doesn't go by the oldest dying first. Unfortunately, Kim's dad Frank was diagnosed with cancer, and my older parents sadly accompanied Kim and me to his funeral. I told you before what a great guy Frank was, and from the hundreds of people who attended his funeral to say good-bye to him, apparently a whole lot of other people felt the same way.

Kim visits his grave on Father's Day. We are lucky because the gravesite is only about a ten-minute walk from where we live. In the meantime, I return each year to San Jose to spend that weekend with my dad to celebrate Father's Day and his birthday, which is also in June. This year, my dad will be eighty-two years old, and he is still going strong. He plans to drive to Los Angeles to sing "Happy Birthday" to Aunt Evelyn, his 103-year-old godmother. He always calls her every Thursday, to see how she is doing. And if he doesn't call, she is on the phone the next day, calling to find out why. She is another one who believes in our family motto: "Can do, or at least try."

I don't think too much about this dying stuff. Two of my cousins died from cancer before they were even fifty years old, and one died before he was twenty-five, and then there is Aunt Billie, ready to celebrate birthday #101, and her sister, wonderful Aunt Edna, who just died at 105 years of age a couple of years ago.

When we were young, my parents talked to me and my brothers and sister about death, because they considered themselves older parents. They wanted us to know to whom we would go to live if they died while we were still children. When we shared this information with our friends in the neighborhood, it made them a little uncomfortable. Some people don't like talking about death, I guess.

Our parents made sure we knew and liked the people we were

to go live with. They put in their will that we would live with the great Uncle Stew and Aunt Peggy, who lived in Maryland. Uncle Stew had a lovely house, big enough to hold all of us, and he owned a bright yellow Porsche car that he called his yellow bird. On their twenty-fifth wedding anniversary, Mom and I surprised him and Aunt Peggy by flying to Maryland for the big celebration they were having. The next day I helped him rotate the tires on that yellow bird. After helping him with that, he told my mom that he knew I was a "can do" kid.

Once we settled that dying issue (that God was in charge of it), all we had to do was just get on with living our busy, happy, and interesting family life. As Mira, my four-year-old godchild, used to say, "It's an adventure." And I thought, *You got that right!*

The timing on this move worked well for Jason, Kim, and me. Kim and I got married in August, and the lease on my apartment ended in September. That gave Jason and me enough time to clean and clear the apartment, so no fees would be added. That is why I always make sure I pay my rent on time, so I do not have to pay any late fees.

Jason's parents had just built a new home near Santa Maria and would be moving down there in September. He was planning to move in with another friend of his near his parents' new home. Yes, this was working out just fine for everyone involved. I reminded Mom to change my address at the post office because I did not want to miss getting any of my mail, especially my *Wrestling* magazine.

Kim and I decided to use my bedroom furniture and her living room furniture, and we put my sofa bed in the extra bedroom of our two-bedroom apartment. We would use that extra room as a combination guest room/office for our computers and a desk for taking care of our bills and other business. There was a big closet where I put my file box for receipts and papers, extra bed linens, and my small safe with a special combination lock.

We used our family pictures and artwork for decorating. My mother-in-law Judy is a great decorator and has loads of good ideas for making a house look really pretty and comfortable. We put family pictures all over the place. We could look around and smile at our parents, our siblings, and especially our cute little nieces and nephews. They were always smiling right back at us. Our home was and is a happy place to be.

Since we set our stuff up in the apartment that Kim was already leasing, I just needed to go into the office and add my name to the lease. It would have been nice if we could have gotten a new apartment, so I would not always feel like I was living in "Kim's place," but a really nice place at a reasonable price is not that easy to find in California.

And this apartment was in a great location. It was just two blocks from the grocery store, five blocks from our bank, two blocks from many restaurants and shopping centers, and only about a mile from another Michaels store, where I had already applied for a new job and had been accepted. One mile was an easy walk for me, and of course I could always take a bus if the weather was bad. Kim could walk about two blocks and catch the bus to her new job. We always purchase a monthly bus pass, just in case we need it. The city of Santa Maria has recently created a nice addition to the bus pass rules. You do not have to get a new one every month as before, when sometimes you had not used all the funds on it. Now we can use the pass until our rides have consumed all the money on it.

Some of the added attractions at the apartment complex included a swimming pool (Kim and I both liked to swim), a weight room, a tennis court, and easy parking for our visitors. I could not complain, even if it meant 'moving into Kim's place.' Besides that, my Section 8 housing approval from Santa Clara County was accepted at this place, so we were able to afford the rent on our own income.

I had made arrangements back in June to start working at the Santa Maria Michaels store in September, a few days after my birthday. It was mostly a matter of transferring my records from the Sunnyvale store to the Santa Maria store. I had a good work record (hard worker, seldom absent, never late, pleasant attitude, and willing to work early or do overtime if I was needed).

Kim had worked at the Roadhouse Grill restaurant before we married. We enjoyed going there for the good food and seeing her former co-workers. The Grill provided free peanuts, and it was fun to follow their tradition of throwing the empty peanut shells on the floor. From the Grill it was easy to get to a nearby theatre to see many of our favorite movies. My dad's mother, Grandma Gert, would not have liked the Grill, because she always loved to keep her home nice and neat and clean.

Whenever Grandma came to visit us when I was a little kid, we had to clean our rooms with extra special care. Mom would say, "The white glove is coming." They had learned to say the "white glove is coming" when my dad was in the Army. When they moved from one military housing complex to another, someone would really come by and check that they had cleaned everything thoroughly. They thought that the inspector wore white gloves. Anyway, we kids worked very hard, because we really wanted to please Grandma.

Besides funds that our pay checks provided, Kim was receiving a small amount of Supplemental Security Income (SSI) funds, and I was getting a small amount of money from my dad's Social Security benefits, called SSA funds. So we were able to pay our bills and save a little for a vacation and weekend fun. We both liked to go to live entertainment shows, and we do whenever we get a chance. Although my paychecks are deposited directly to my bank account, I like going in and doing my other banking business. Of course, I just use my ATM card to get my weekly cash allowance, or to buy special cards or gifts for my two families. By just taking out my weekly spending allowance on Monday's, I avoid overspending on treats, games and food.

People are often amazed that I know all of my banking account numbers without looking at my checks. The tellers at the bank often greet me by name, and one tells us that she loves it when I come to her window, because she knows that all the information will be properly filled in on my deposit or withdrawal slips, and that my checks will be endorsed with correct name and numbers. She says that it is amazing how often she has to add a "date" for others, and she has to ask them to add their account numbers on their slips.

By the way, having a savings account is okay when you are getting SSA funds, but you cannot have much savings if you receive SSI funds. We later learned that while the SSI program is run by the Social Security Administration, it is not Social Security funding. Social Security offices just administer the program for the federal government. It is a separate program set up by the federal government to help the poor and disabled. Unfortunately, because it is so hard for them to get employment, many people with disabilities are also poor.

Many people mistakenly think that individuals with disabilities cannot be married and receive SSA funds from their parents' accounts. We learned that someone who is getting SSA funds can be married, but they must be married to someone who also gets SSA funds, and then their funding can continue. But that same person cannot receive their SSA funds if they marry someone who gets SSI funds. My mom has a PhD and she still cannot figure the reasoning behind that rule.

We could understand it, if the rule was whether or not you are married or single. But whether or not you are married to someone getting SSA or SSI funding as the rule makes no sense at all. It does seem that we can sometimes create confusing rules, where they are not needed, and they make very little sense to most people. I hope that by the time you are reading this, someone will at least be working on getting this straightened out. The way it is now, it can prevent persons with disabilities from getting married and having a very happy, productive life. You don't think that is the reason they have that rule do you? Maybe President Obama will be able to put this on his list next, to fix it for individuals with disabilities. I suppose someone needs to let him know about it.

Kim and I share the cost of living, paying the bills, and doing the housework. Being a bachelor for about five years, I had plenty of experience washing and drying my clothes, cleaning the bathroom, vacuuming, fixing my meals, and paying the bills. I set up savings and checking accounts at the same bank Kim was using. We have kept our accounts separate (just like my parents, and they have been happily married over fifty years). You got that right-- I figured it could work for us, since it had worked so well for them.

We each pay our part of the bills from our own checkbook. For example, I would write a check for $500 and she would write a check for $500 and we would go to the office to pay our $1,000 lease when we lived in Kim's apartment. Every month, Kim's mom would tally up our checkbooks to be sure we were keeping an accurate account of what funds we were using and what our balances were. Being the CEO of a company, she watches our balances to the penny.

Being married was similar to living with my roommate Jason, except Jason and I had separate rooms, and we were not in love.

Kim and I decided that we did not want children, so she used birth control pills. Unfortunately, that caused her to gain weight, so I agreed to have a vasectomy. My surgery went well, and we got a chance to stay at my parents' home (since my mom is a nurse) for about five days, just to be sure everything was okay. Kim and I even enjoyed breakfast in bed one morning. "Just a little special treat," Mom said. Kim totally loved it! Both of our parents enjoy doing nice little things for us, including buying us souvenirs whenever they take trips.

Speaking of my surgery, we soon realized that I needed to get a primary care doctor down in Santa Maria who was closer than my doctors in San Jose. It was not the easiest job. We talked to family members and friends to get references and suggestions. We finally found a wonderful doctor, Dr. D. He and his sister, who is a physician assistant, take very good care of me. Actually, they take good care of me and Kim and all the immediate members of her family. They all switched to my doctor after they saw what good care he gave me, and their doctor was getting older and about ready to retire.

I decided to use the same dentist Kim's family was using, as well as the same podiatrist that Kim used. I still go to Kaiser Permanente in San Jose for an annual physical and every two years to get my eyes checked and my glasses upgraded there.

When I got back to work after my vasectomy surgery, I found my work hours at Michaels were getting less and less. My job coach and I started looking for another job. I landed a great job at a local fast food restaurant. I do everything in there excluding the cash register and cooking. I take the orders from the computer screen and fill them on trays, I refill the soda machines, clean the bathrooms, clean the tables, change the liners in the trash cans, sweep the floor, take orders to folks at the drive through, and any other little thing that I can do to help my coworkers.

Of course, I take care of any special requests our customers ask for. Most of the time, I say, "Oh sure," or "That's just fine," or "Sure, I can get that." They do not hesitate to call on me if they have a question or a problem. I stay busy all the time I am at work. I have received very good evaluations from, the manager. And she is good about giving me days off if I need to go to San Jose for special occasions or to go on vacation with my new family. She asked if I wanted to learn to use the cash register, but I said, "I can do without the stress of those long lines at lunch time." They are very pleased with my work, and three years ago, I received an award for five years of employment. The district manager said he anxiously waits to give me my ten-year pin. I will be excited to get it too.

A filmmaker who was creating a documentary on individuals with disabilities in the workforce got permission from the restaurant management (and from me, of course) to film me at work, just going about my usual work routine. Was it a little added excitement? You bet! Someday you may see the film on one of your local PBS television stations.

While they were setting up their camera equipment, I noticed that their electrical cord was blocking customers from some tables, and the cord could also trip a customer. I immediately showed them another place where they could plug in their equipment.

My mom was watching me and told the district manager what I was doing: my thoughtfulness, my keen observations, and my self-confidence to take action about what I saw. He assured her that he knew what a great employee he had.

The film producer then followed me home to get a few scenes of Kim and me in our condo. She wanted to get some shots of us going about our daily routines. Actually, that was the second time I had been filmed going about my daily routines. A lady from New York was making a movie about a young man with Down syndrome. She was excited about the demonstration video we sent. She called a few times to say that she really liked the video, but the producer was very busy. She said it would take a while to get back to me. I have not heard anything since those calls. I do know that the movie has not been made. Who knows, I may still be doing some modeling and movie work one day. I am still interested.

People seem very interested in videotapes of me working, but I hope one day they will do a video of me at the voting booth. I like to discuss the people running for office and the issues on the ballot with my family, and then I decide how I want to vote. Sometimes, I decide that the issue is just too complicated for me to make a decision, so I do not vote on those things. I remember that Mom was very excited when Barack Obama ran for president, but I liked Hillary Clinton, so Hillary it was for me. Sometimes, my Aunt Terrie drives me to the voting place. If it is not too far from my house, of course, I just walk to the polls.

I feel that this voting thing is very important. I fill out the ballot at home, so it does not take much time when I go in to vote. As James Brown would say, "I feel good," and I feel proud when I cast my vote.

Of course, after moving from San Jose to another part of California, I needed to get acquainted with the same kinds of agencies that had helped me set up my independent lifestyle in Sunnyvale. I got a new case manager at the Tri-Counties Regional

Center, signed up at the Vocational Technical Center for job assistance, contacted the State Department of Rehabilitation, and enrolled with an agency called Lifesteps to get the same type of services provided to me by Greater Opportunities up in the San Jose area.

Once you are familiar with how these different agencies work, it is easy to handle the changes. It is just a matter of getting acquainted with new faces—new people doing the same type of assistance for you. I have been very lucky; all the helpers I left in Santa Clara County were just fine, and now all my helpers in Santa Barbara County are just fine also. There is one thing that has not changed: my parents are still my great conservators, no matter where I live. Part of being smart enough for living independently, is being open to knowing when to let others help you. My parents still come to my annual meeting with all of the agencies that work with me, to help me report on how I am doing and decide on next year's goals.

Mom and Dad are thinking about adding my brothers and sister to this conservator job. They will need to go to court to add them on as conservators. It is nice, having my good friend Pete as my attorney (no pay needed), and having my family members as my conservators. Without the conservator title, my parents could not get my doctors, dentist, or other agencies working with me to share my information and tests results with them. Once a client is eighteen years old, these agencies are not obligated to include the parents in their meetings or decisions. So it would just be the agency staff making decisions about my life. Sometimes it is illegal for them to share information (even with parents, if they are not conservators) about someone who is over eighteen years old, no matter what their physical or mental condition is. I don't want to make big decisions without my family's help—you got that right! Why, even my smart sister and brothers often 'check in' with mom and dad on big decisions also.

I had a chance to see some of my former helpers back in Santa Clara County when I returned to receive a Valley of Hearts'

Independent Living Award. I wanted them to know some of what I have learned about living independently. I like people to know that although I do not talk a lot, it is easy for me to figure things out and find answers in my head. For example, I figured out that when other people are not making phone calls to me, that probably means that they do not want frequent calls from me. So I do not bug them with calls. But I am really happy to take their calls when they have time. Besides that, I have very good memory skills, and once I learn something or I am told something, I got it. Why, I even call Dad every September 9 to remind him that it's his mother's birthday, even though she died nine years ago. I know he likes to go and put flowers on her grave on special days. It is not hard for me to handle living independently, but it was nice of them to give me an award for it.

Can you believe it? I have worked long enough to receive Social Security financial assistance (SSA funds) from my own work record. And I still receive a small amount of funds from my dad's Social Security account. Kim had been receiving Supplemental Security Income (SSI) assistance, but since the death of her father, she gets SSA from his Social Security account. This helps us a lot because SSA provides more funds and puts less restrictions on what we can have financially, or what we can own or do.

Our parents still provide us with some funds to help with special things like purchasing our Jenny Craig food. Kim and I are both trying to lose some weight. They also help with the cost of our exercise program at the workout center and our major vacations.

We have great fun when our godchild Mira and our other nephews, nieces, and their parents drive down for a visit during summer vacation or for my birthday. If we don't go out to a restaurant, we throw a party right in our condo. The kids enjoy the playground and the pool. By using my den and our guest room, there is usually plenty of room for everyone, although it gets a bit crowded at the breakfast table.

By the way, having a godchild lets us feel like parents, without having that big responsibility. That was a very special and happy day for Kim and me when we participated in Mira's christening. I am really grateful to my sister Jill and her husband for giving us this honor. Now I am a kind of father and Kim is a kind of mother.

If there is grilling or barbecue to be prepared for a gathering, we can always count on our very best friend Patti. She's a great cook, and she is also willing to give us a manicure or a pedicure now and then, as a special treat. We can talk to her about anything and everything. She loves and respects us, and she helps us figure stuff out. We can get advice from her without feeling like we are going to our parents for everything.

Kim and I moved into this nice three-bedroom condo last year. It is within easy walking distance of our bank, grocery store, drugstores, and so much more. My other mother, my mother-in-law Judy, did a great job finding this place for us. All of our new Santa Maria health care providers—doctors, dentist, podiatrist, are nearby.

Our families are still doing a great job of sharing us for holidays and special events. For example, if we spend Thanksgiving in San Jose, we spend Christmas in Santa Maria, and the following year we reverse that. Family members all take turns driving us from and to San Jose and Santa Maria. They often do an exchange of us at a point half way between San Jose and Santa Maria. The exit is easy for Dad to remember, it is Canal Street. Everyone from New Orleans knows that famous Canal Street name.

Both of our families share in major celebrations and activities. While Judy, Kim, and I went to Oakland for Aunt Evelyn's (my dad's aunt and godmother) hundredth birthday party, my parents came to Santa Maria for Kim's grandmother's ninetieth birthday bash. And last year, when Judy remarried; we all got together for her wonderful wedding to Jimmy. I now have a new father-in-law, and he is quite a guy. He keeps us laughing all the time with his interesting stories.

It all kind of brings me back to that Corky Riley television show: yes indeed, *life goes on.* And on, and on, and on …

This is Dean A. A. Poyadue saying to the world, "You can just call me Dean, and don't rain on my parade."

So long!

EPILOGUE   A WORD FROM MY MOM

It's always so nice to have a little dessert to top off a really good meal, and that sweet morsel is even more delightful and welcomed after a not-so-great culinary attempt. For those of you who have just finished feeding on *Call Me Dean*, this dessert's just for you. I want to give you a brief update on Dean and Kim; share a few more personal insights into Dean's personality and his positive, successful way of being in the world; and then add a few general words about individuals with special needs living independently. The latter part will also touch on parents learning to let go and changes that have occurred in society that make living independently more successful for individuals who just happen to have a special need or disability.

First and foremost, Dean and Kim continue to lead very successful happy lives: living independently in their condo, working part time, and participating fully in both of their families' activities and celebrations. They have a part-time house cleaner who comes by twice a month to give their place a good going over; otherwise they take care of everything (from taking out the trash to bringing in the mail), and they do a very good job of it. They continue to handle their business: doing their banking, making a grocery list, shopping, and paying their bills just like the rest of us who try to keep a good credit score.

Like so many of us in America, they battle the bulge through extra exercise (walking, swimming, going to the YMCA, and using personal trainers from time to time) and listening to Diane, their wonderful personal counselor.. Their home is always a warm and welcoming place for visiting family members and friends. They pride themselves on being gracious host and hostess, and it shows through as they give you a tour of their home and offer you some liquid refreshment. They do such a good job of being host and hostess, that I always put them in charge of that job at my annual Christmas Eve Spaghetti Feast. At this time they are anxiously planning how they will celebrate their tenth anniversary together. They are strongly considering taking a cruise, which they both enjoy. All in all, to borrow a favorite phrase of Dean's, they are doing just fine.

Speaking of Dean, I often ask myself, "Is there a difference between unique and special?" Because he has such good judgment skills and such an emotionally balanced way of being in the world, while fully using his level of intelligence that I often want to say that he is unique. But I believe he is unique only when compared to just any human being in this world. I do not believe he is unique as a very rare capable person who has Down syndrome or some other disability. I know there are many such persons in our society who are capable, and there are others who, if given the chance, could function just as well as Dean and Kim.

Dean tends to live in the present. That is something emotional gurus often try to teach the rest of us to do. They insist we will be much happier if we learn to live in the present and not keep returning to the past or jumping ahead to the future. I often tell parents of children with special needs, "Do not cross tomorrow's bridges of sorrow today, for tomorrow they may no longer be." Because Dean seems to automatically choose to live in the present, he is a happier person (most of the time.) Because he is happy, those around him also tend to be in a pretty good mood.

Dean never interrupts when others are talking. If you have a conversation with him, and the two of you spontaneously start to talk at the same moment in the lull of a conversation, I promise you he will be the first to say, "No, no, you go ahead." I have never seen it fail, no matter to whom he is chatting, including me.

Because he doesn't interrupt, and because he knows he must follow your words carefully to be sure he understands you correctly, he looks at you and he tends to be a very good listener. I believe at least half of the world is looking for a good listener—someone who truly hears them; therefore, others like to be in his presence.

One day while we were having lunch at the restaurant where Dean works, one of the customers was talking to me about the old gentleman she was caring for. She whispered, "He is grumpy all day, except when he is here being served by your son. When he gets home, he is still smiling and saying nice things about his encounter with him."

Yes, Dean, you are doing your part in that circle of life where one who receives help, also ends up giving help; you are taking your turn at helping as you hoped you would be able to do someday. That includes helping, not only this old gentleman, but also the young gardener at your condo complex, who is going back to college because he said that he was inspired by the good example he sees you setting every day as you head out to work on time, well groomed, carrying your satchel, and ready to take on life's challenges.

Dean does not overanalyze things. I believe he sees life as important but not so serious. Little problems do not become major issues or blown out of proportion, because he does not pick them apart. He accepts them as problems, at their own low level of concern, and he immediately goes into problem-solving mode.

While he does not overly analyze, he is quite the thinker; for example, the staff at the weight control center had moved their offices across town. I had mailed Dean's payment to them, but the post office sent it back to me. I told Dean that I would put it in another envelope with their new address. He immediately suggested to me, "Mom, send letter to me, I give to Diane." I agreed, and I now always send that letter, and often other things, to him to handle. As he says, "My address not changing." Being a rather typical modern day kid, of course, he always asks how I plan to replace his funds if he pays a bill that I promised I would take care of

As another example, his in-laws scheduled a wonderful vacation trip to Kentucky. Two days before they were to catch the plane (even with all the packing and excitement going on), he called, "Mom, change doctor's date for foot care." His mother-in-law had changed their return day, and the new date was after his appointment. "Yes, Dean. I will," I said. Two days into the vacation, I got a call, "Did you change doctor date?" he asked. "Oops, no, I did not," I said, "but I will, right this minute."

While visiting him and his wife, I drove him to work and then went back to their home to spend a little more time with Kim before his dad and I hit the road to head back to San Jose. His dad and I dropped in for lunch at his place of work before starting our four-hour drive home. While waiting for our order, he dropped by our table and asked, "Mom, you get gas?" "No," I said, "why?" "I saw gas line low." "Thanks for reminding me," I said. "I did not get any because Dad is planning to fill up the tank after lunch." Dean did not want us running out of gas on the freeway.

These are just a few of hundreds of such incidents. While he is not an over-analyzer, he is a thinking man; not only thinking of dates and schedules and gas gauges, but also thinking about people. Recently he called and asked, "Mom, you call Aunt Shoo-Shoo? TV weather report bad." "Yes Dean," I said, "I called her and Aunt Liz; the tornado was near them, but they are okay." Knowing how it pains his dad for any money to be wasted, he gave the following toast at his sister's wedding: "I would like to give a toast to my sister, Jill. I love you, Jill. Be happy. Now my dad will not have to pay your phone bill." Months before, he had written it exactly as he wanted to deliver it, and that he did to everyone's delight.

And yes, Dean also thinks of his own comfort. Before he got an alarm clock so that he would not have to depend on others to awaken him, more than once he said to me, "Mom, you wake me in the morning, you wake me easy. Dad said he would, but he wakes me rough." He was saving himself the "trauma" of his dad's loud knocks on his bedroom door and his booming voice shouting, "Up, up, up!"

As his ten-year-old nephew Aidan says adamantly, "Uncle Dean is not special needs; you can discuss anything with him. He just has a speech problem." Yes, Aidan, he tends to have that effect on people. I remember when I took him to see a doctor visiting from Germany, who often worked with children who have Down syndrome. The doctor's first question to me was, "Does *he* have a problem?" I said, "Yes, he has Down syndrome." I don't know how scientifically true it is, but he said, "Oh," and then added, "Not many babies of African heritage are born with Downs."

When a passer-by says, "Hi Dean," it makes Dean feel high on life, high on himself, and high on the speaker. If someone passes by and does not speak to him, he usually says, "He didn't see me." With that non-blaming attitude, he remains content, and that flows to the next person he meets. He is accepting of others and therefore comfortable with himself. Or perhaps, because he is comfortable with himself, he is accepting of others. For example, when his barber learned he was getting married, she promised him a free haircut for his wedding day. Of course he told her, "That's just fine." And he insisted on me giving her a generous tip.

As Dean has written, "I am special because I like myself, and I got a family who loves me." Perhaps more of us should learn to like ourselves and let family members know that we love them; just maybe, we would all treat each other a little better and have that "kinder, gentler world" President Bush #43 promised us. We wouldn't all immediately become a Mother Teresa, but we might at least become a Dean.

Dean does not have to practice being humble, he just is. When it comes to doing chores, he seems to function on the principle, "If I have time to do it, then I am not doing too much. I am not doing more than my share." That holds true whether he is at work or at home. If he is busy—folding clothes, playing video games, or watching *World Wrestling Entertainment*—he will tell you so. Until now, I have not heard him say a negative comment about a single person. Dean probably is unique *and* special in that way.

And now, here are a few words in general about transitioning to independent living for individuals with special needs. I recently gave a keynote speech at a conference for parents and professionals entitled - It's Their Life. More and more young adults with special needs are telling their parents that 'it is their life;' they want to have a say in it, and they want a full circle of life's experiences and relationships. Yes, it is their life, but as parents, boy, are we in it! And we are in it because it is not only their life, but their life is on the line.

If we look at this scenario as a movie, the young person with special needs would be the main character, his or her parents would be the supporting cast, and the professionals involved would be the producers and directors. Each of them has specific roles to play and duties to perform to help prepare the young individual for independent living: their health care, their education, their jobs, and so on.

Like most young people, the main character's role consists of going to school, studying, doing homework, maintaining physical health, exercising, and working with the parents and professionals who are involved in his or her growth and development. It may seem like a simple and easy part to play, but it is very important and key to the success of this transition to independent living. Then add to this, their need to face the fears and challenges that scare all young people as they embark on adult life responsibilities and leaving their parents' safe, comfortable nest. This truly is the biggest job of all.

As supporting characters, parents have several major jobs to do. One of those jobs, of course, is learning to let go. That is huge, that is scary, and it is ongoing. As my own mother said, as she let go of her brood of eleven, "I let go and let God." Later, I will share a brief article I wrote when Dean was about nine years old, as I realized that I was learning to let go, even at that young age. I encourage parents to start early to learn to let go.

Parents then take on six major roles (they become the CIA and the SSS):

C: Case manager: keeping records, calendaring meetings, making appointments.

I: Information provider: share family, health, and education histories, and current events.

A: Advocate (provide a voice for): helping the main character access services; in this role, parents need to learn the difference between being assertive and being aggressive. *Assertive* people speak up for their issue, but do not disrespect or attack the person to whom they are talking. They learn to start most of their sentences with the little word "I." *Aggressive* people also speak up for their issue but have no regard for the other person; they often attack and thus alienate them by starting their sentences with "You."

S: Set priorities when decisions are being made (consulting the main character).

S: Select housing preference/living arrangements in consultation with the main character.

S: Support the other players on the team as a supporting link, linking things and people together.

The professionals (the producers and directors) have major roles in preparing the main character for his or her role and in managing the agencies that serve and support the main character. They also must take on the CIA jobs. And both they and the parents must understand and follow the laws of the land (local, state, and federal). It helps tremendously if these partners know something about collaborating, because that is what they must do.

That collaboration process should at least include the following simple formula that I call collaborating mathematically: "Come together to *add* each other's expertise in order to decide on what the problem is and to create a plan for solving it. *Subtract* their differences for the time being and utilize the things they can agree on. *Divide* the work. And thus *multiply* their successes, by not caring who gets the credit."

People involved in collaborating with others should not lose sight of the fact that most decisions will function like a mobile: any decision you make will not only cause that one piece of the mobile to move, the action will also cause all of the other pieces to move and be affected by that piece's motion. Life's decisions are like a child's mobile. Our lives are so interconnected now that this process happens not only in one's personal life, but also in agencies, institutions, and global governmental decisions. The key is to be aware of this phenomenon and adjust your plans and decisions accordingly. Just being aware of this helps you to make wiser decisions in the first place.

When collaborating, openly state your agreement whenever others (even those seen as the opposition) say something with which you do agree: "I like what Harry just said." "I agree with Helen on that point." Then when you do have to voice opposition, the others are more likely to listen. One last negotiation point: when the other side says "no;" take it as an opening for further discussion. You might say something like "I can see I have not made myself clear."

How does a parent, conservator, or other family member prepare for the role of case manager? I think most of us just grow into it, as more and more things land on our plates to handle. Start by keeping one comprehensive calendar for everything, even potential events. Another thing that helps me is making copies of the paperwork (not only one, but sometimes two). If you can, purchase a copier, it will be well worth the savings and headaches of having to go out and pay for copies. Many computer printers now allow you to make copies as well (and send faxes too.) I feel less anxious knowing that there is more than one copy available, if a document is lost or misfiled. I figure the odds are in my favor for finding it if there is more than just the original floating around somewhere. Using a two- to four-drawer file cabinet encourages good case management habits. My general basic rule is, "When in doubt, don't, don't throw it out."

I also encourage parents of children with special needs (or anyone responsible for someone else's welfare) to use a briefcase to carry important papers to meetings. Besides making it easier to have what you need all in one place, psychologically it seems that coming into a meeting with your briefcase boosts your confidence level and often generates more respect from the group. When you enter the meeting room, keep your head up and stride to a seat in the middle of the long side of the meeting table. It will provide you with the power of access to more of the participants, and it is a great spot from which to be seen and heard by all, as you use assertive, nonaggressive language to make your child's case.

Parents might want to start thinking early in their child's life about preparing themselves and their child for letting go. I wrote the following article for the Parents Helping Parents Newsletter, Special Addition, about twenty-six years ago, when Dean was nine years old. Maybe Dean did get an early start, and perhaps that has played a part in his living independent successfully. I hope "Letting Go" will give other parents the tiny push they may need to nudge them in the right direction to accomplish their child's goal.

Letting Go

As I dropped Dean off at the people-cluttered gates of his latest elementary school, a slight pang of anxiety hit me as I watched him deliberately dawdle off, wave, throw a kiss to me, and then disappear among the crowd of school children. Hesitantly, I forced myself to put the car into gear and drove off, thinking, *how hard it is letting go.*

When I began to remember all the schools, professionals, and situations that Dean had handled, a fast swelling pride began to nudge my anxiety aside. I, like so many parents of children with special needs, had to start letting go of this child so much sooner.

By age two to three months, he was being given over to an infant educator about twice a week.

Pride grew as I realized that in nine years he had learned to negotiate eight different schools; each year having to make new friends and adjust to a whole cadre of new professionals. How much more we families, and society, often expect from these little ones who are supposedly less endowed. My two normal "genius" children have had the security of walking just two blocks to the same school for the past eight years—not starting at two months of age, but three years—secure in their ability to communicate their needs, wants, pains, or joys with clear, articulate words. Not so Dean.

As the traffic light turned red, I thought back to the day before, when my normal sixteen-year-old son, Keith, overheard Dean working intensely on his math and phonics. He said, "Mom, you know, if those Down's kids had a good brain, there wouldn't be anything they couldn't do."

"What do you men?" I asked.

"Look how hard he works, he tries, and tries with such persistence and patience, he would be able to do almost anything he attempted."

I had to agree, and I sensed a little guilt in Keith for perhaps not using "the good brain" he has, as well as he might.

I hope Keith will let go any guilt and instead take on Dean as an "effort" role model. Oh! The light is green. My thoughts go on to my daughter Jill jokingly complaining about Dean, "Mom, he is just too darn polite." He seldom forgets to say, "Thank you, Mommy."

"No, Jill," I said, "Society demands more politeness from those who are different, be they handicapped or ethnic minorities. They must be a little less noisy, a little less conspicuous, a little less obtrusive, and yes, a little more polite."

—Florene

In the almost thirty-five years since Dean was born, many

things have changed in our world that help individuals with special needs, senior citizens, and many others to live more independently than they might otherwise be able to. We—parents, professionals, service systems, governmental institutions, legal entities, and the general public—have all come a long way in just the past fifteen years in our understanding of the "abilities" of individuals with disabilities; these individuals, I think, always knew how capable they were.

I believe particular developments not only contributed to Dean's ability to transition to independence, but also allowed it to speed along, flourish, thrive, and take root, becoming just an ordinary expectation, not a unique phenomenon. Aside from his own innate abilities and great decision-making skills, Dean's transition to independent living has been fueled by changes mainly in the following five arenas: parent empowerment, society's attitude toward differences, governmental and disability-related nonprofit organizations, technology, and Taft, a community college in California.

Parent-to-parent self-help programs like Parents Helping Parents (PHP) create empowered parents as equal collaborating partners at the decision-making table, and we also give each other the courage to let our children go, to face the world. These parent-to-parent self-help programs not only provide emotional support, so that parents have the strength and spirit to seek a better way, they also become training schools for parents and professionals to learn about the laws that protect the rights of these citizens, their children with special needs. PHP is also a PTI (Parent Training and Information Center).There are parent-to-parent centers in most of our fifty states; they have become the central hub where families find answers, services, and resources. They are family empowerment centers.

These programs even train physicians in better ways of breaking bad diagnostic news to parents. Done wrong, it could cause a huge gap in the parent-child bonding process. They encourage industries to create assistive technology to aid their children, and they confront the legal system and encourage judges to take a second look at how kids with learning disabilities are treated in juvenile halls.

They work hand in hand with local universities to better prepare those entering the new disability-inclusive educational classroom. They fight to enhance collaboration and interaction between the many helping professionals serving their children, so their children can have better care through a more coordinated system of services. Many professionals were not taught collaboration in their formal training, therefore they are not used to sharing information about their clients and/or other professionals serving that client. Empowered parents lead to more empowered children and a belief that they not only can handle being in the community, they belong in the community, and have a right to be there. These individuals with special needs can spread kindness, caring, and compassion, which this world never has too much of.

Society's attitude toward individuals with disabilities has been transformed through programs such as Special Olympics, Buddy Walks, Sibling Workshops, Children's Neighborhood Integration, and integrated theatrical productions. Society's eyes have been opened to truly see the capabilities of all our citizens, and that has fostered not only tolerance; but also acceptance, and soon appreciation, of a wonderful, contributing sector of society they had long neglected getting to know. That change has been another key for unlocking the chains of isolation and separation of individuals with disabilities from the rest of society, often housing them in institutions "for their own good," we often said.

Spending time with individuals with disabilities is the quickest and easiest way to get rid of anger, fear, or stereotypical thinking about others who are different. When was last time you had someone with a different racial background, religious preference, sexual orientation, or disability at your home for dinner? Try it; you might not only learn something, you might make a really good friend, and you just might like it. Almost more important than that, what a beneficial example for your children who are present!

You can help spare the next generation the pains of pre-judging (pains for the judger and the judged).

Much has changed in the last twenty-five years, thanks to the US government and nonprofit adult disability rights advocacy organizations such as the Disability Rights Education Defense Fund. The wheels of progress for inclusion and independence started rolling mightily in 1975 (happily, the same year of Dean's birth) with the passage of Public Law 94-142. That law provided individuals with disabilities the right to a free, appropriate education, in the least restricted (integrated) environment. Finally, children with disabilities became visible in classrooms and on playgrounds across the country, for other children, teachers, and the public to see. Inclusion was finally started then, and is now here to stay. Finally, they too had a right to go to school and learn.

During the 1980s and 1990s, at Surgeon General C. Everett Koop's annual health conferences, we sang about family-centered, community-based, culturally competent, coordinated care. We not only sang, we—parents, professionals, and our government—worked together across the country to make this better way of care happen. For Dean, it is here, and I hope, for many others, if not now, soon. We must all continue to work as individuals and in groups to create the community, the America, the world we want, not only for individuals with special needs, but for all of us—a world that is caring, ethical, and fair for all.

It is a readily accepted conclusion that technology plays a significant role in almost every aspect of a person's ability (whether ill, old, or disabled) to successfully transition to more independent living. From the cell phone to the very welcomed GPS to guide us where we are headed, we would not want to be without these technological advances. Technology aids us in our personal care, mobility, transportation, communication, safety, cooking, and other ways too numerous to mention here.

From low tech to high tech, we continue to sing the praises of technology. If you have not done so already, I encourage you to visit a Special Tech Center near you. Apple Computer played a significant role in helping to get Special Tech Centers up and running across the country; we at PHP thank them for their great contribution to our Introduction to Technology Easing Children's Handicaps (ITECH) – an assistive technology center. The tech center serves children with special needs, also their families, other students, and professionals in the community.

By far, the most significant change that had the greatest impact on Dean's transition success was Taft Junior College's two-year, comprehensive transition program called Transition to Independent Living (TIL). You name it, they taught it there (budgets, travel, housekeeping, cooking, specific jobs for potential gainful employment, relationship skills, how to include fun in your life, knowing the difference between needing something and just wanting it, safety, and many other things including reading, writing, and arithmetic. And the students had the wonderful experience of living away from their homes, in dorms on campus. Dean met his wife Kim there, and they continue to enjoy going back for periodic reunions held by the school. I strongly feel that there should be a Taft style TIL program in every county—at the least, one in every state of our great union.

At a recent conference called "It's Their Life," we all agreed on the following unofficial Bill of Rights for young adults with special needs/disabilities:

Bill of Rights for Individuals with Disabilities

Every person has the right to:
1. Be treated with respect and dignity, to have others see and not ignore them.
2. Have privacy and the opportunity to participate in society.
3. Be free of physical and mental abuse.
4. Refuse certain treatments.
5. Have a "personal love interest."
6. Be informed about and involved in their home location.

7. Manage their financial affairs (according to their ability).
8. Know what services will be provided and when to expect them.
9. Expect safe and competent care/services.
10. Confidential treatment of their records and papers.
11. Receive advance notice before being moved.
12. Have a conservator to assist as needed, just as some folks have attorneys or accountants. So please do not call it "being conserved." This takes the burden of final decisions off of service agencies when it is not necessary.
13. Last, but not least, everyone should have the right to risk.

Most of us take risks every day: driving the freeway, catching a plane, taking new drugs on the shelf, and so on. This last "right to risk" reminds me of part of a poem I wrote many years ago, in reference to our children with special needs:

> Like birds in a gilded cage—safe.
> Protected, but not free.
> Even they long to flee,
> And face the world's adversity.

Teacher Pat was right, Dean: Oh, the Places You Will Go! You have traveled from Hawaii to Washington, DC, from Canada to Kentucky, and many points between. You were a big hit when you escorted your mom to her first high school reunion back in Lovejoy, Illinois. You handled yourself well at national conferences, sitting in the front row seats. And yes, you were there, although I am sure you do not remember it, when Dad took you to see the United States land its first spacecraft on land instead of water. And Dean, as you have so poignantly taught us, although one may not remember all that happens to them, it is a part of them, and influences who and how they are in the world.

Thanks, Dean, for doing your part of helping, which I know is so important to you. And thank you for helping me to learn that: We can waste our lives complaining about the unchosen path we've been handed, or we can choose to rise to the challenge, as we realize that it is not so much about "having" a good day as it is about "making" it a great day for yourself and those around you.

Love, Mom

TODAY, AS ALWAYS

(For son Turhan)

One day flows into another,
Offering sameness, yet difference flutters among the wet green
grass
As we hold on fast to reason and
Embark on another trip.

Life fills our bellies with hors d'oeuvres of stranger friends.
And bids us listen to unseen thoughts and laughter.
As we embark on yet another trip.

We ride the train of life
Today, as always
Alert as hopping rabbits,
Or halted and intrigued as a deer head-lighted.
And yet, we embark on another trip.
—Florene Stewart Poyadue

Open Book Editions
A Berrett-Koehler Partner

Open Book Editions is a joint venture between Berrett-Koehler Publishers and Author Solutions, the market leader in self-publishing. There are many more aspiring authors who share Berrett-Koehler's mission than we can sustainably publish. To serve these authors, Open Book Editions offers a comprehensive self-publishing opportunity.

A Shared Mission

Open Book Editions welcomes authors who share the Berrett-Koehler mission—Creating a World That Works for All. We believe that to truly create a better world, action is needed at all levels—individual, organizational, and societal. At the individual level, our publications help people align their lives with their values and with their aspirations for a better world. At the organizational level, we promote progressive leadership and management practices, socially responsible approaches to business, and humane and effective organizations. At the societal level, we publish content that advances social and economic justice, shared prosperity, sustainability, and new solutions to national and global issues.

Open Book Editions represents a new way to further the BK mission and expand our community. We look forward to helping more authors challenge conventional thinking, introduce new ideas, and foster positive change.

For more information, see the Open Book Editions website: http://www.iuniverse.com/Packages/OpenBookEditions.aspx

Join the BK Community! See exclusive author videos, join discussion groups, find out about upcoming events, read author blogs, and much more! http://bkcommunity.com/